A DENTAL PRACTITIONER H
SERIES EDITED BY DONALD D. DERRICK

CYSTS OF THE ORAL REGIONS

MERVYN SHEAR

D.SC. (DENT.), M.D.S., M.R.C.PATH., H.DIP.DENT., F.O.S. (S.A.).

Professor of Oral Pathology and Head of the Department of Oral Pathology in the School of Pathology of the University of the Witwatersrand and the South African Institute for Medical Research, Johannesburg, South Africa

BRISTOL : JOHN WRIGHT & SONS LTD
1976

ISBN 0 7236 0420 7

PRINTED IN GREAT BRITAIN BY HENRY LING LTD., A SUBSIDIARY OF JOHN WRIGHT & SONS LTD., AT THE DORSET PRESS, DORCHESTER

PREFACE

CYSTS of the jaws and mouth have been recognized as clinical problems for a long time. During the past few years, however, there have been a large number of publications on the subject, reflecting a great increase in interest in the causes, pathogenesis, behaviour, diagnosis and treatment of the various types of cyst.

This book was written in an attempt to record, in one volume, current views on these cysts. Clinical data, primarily from my own records, radiological features, discussion on pathogenesis, descriptions of the pathology and brief comments on treatment have been included for each variety. It is hoped that the work will be helpful to undergraduate and postgraduate students, general dental practitioners, surgeons, radiologists and pathologists.

A considerable proportion of this book was written during a sabbatical leave spent in the Department of Oral Pathology, Royal Dental College, Copenhagen, Denmark, and I am extremely grateful to Professor Jens Pindborg, Head of this Department, for so kindly allowing me access to his material and for letting me use some of it for this book. I should also like to record my gratitude to Denmark's National Bank for generously inviting my family and me to live in one of their flats in Nyhavn 18 during our stay in Copenhagen.

In the preparation of this book, I have been very greatly helped by colleagues who have kindly lent me clinical photographs and radiographs of their cases. I am particularly indebted to Professor John Lemmer for allowing me access to the records of the Division of Radiology in his Department of our School of Dentistry. It is a pleasure to acknowledge the very considerable assistance which I have received from members of my Department: especially Mario Altini, Archibald Scott, Janice Croft, Renee Goldstein, Lenah Free, Miriam Nadel and Barbara Marcus, as well as from Marlies Jansen in the Photographic Division of our School.

Johannesburg, 1976.   M.S.

CONTENTS

CONTENTS

INTRODUCTION

A CYST is a pathological cavity having fluid, semifluid or gaseous contents and which is not created by the accumulation of pus (Kramer, 1974). It is frequently, but not always, lined by epithelium.

Numerous classifications have been published of cysts of the jaws. Most of these are perfectly satisfactory and the reader is advised to use any classification which he finds valuable as an aid to memory and understanding. The classification used in this book is modified from the one recommended by the World Health Organization International Reference Centre for the Histological Definition and Classification of Odontogenic Tumours, Jaw Cysts and Allied Lesions (Pindborg and Kramer, 1971).

CLASSIFICATION

I. CYSTS OF THE JAWS

A. Epithelial

1. *Developmental*

(A) ODONTOGENIC

    i. Primordial cyst (keratocyst)

    ii. Gingival cyst of infants

    iii. Gingival cyst of adults

    iv. Lateral periodontal cyst

    v. Dentigerous (follicular) cyst

    vi. Eruption cyst

    vii. Calcifying odontogenic cyst

(B) NON-ODONTOGENIC

    i. Nasopalatine duct (incisive canal) cyst

    *ii. Median palatine, median alveolar and median mandibular cysts

    *iii. Globulomaxillary cyst

    iv. Nasolabial (nasoalveolar) cyst

2. *Inflammatory*

    Radicular cyst

B. Non-epithelial

1. Simple bone cyst (traumatic, haemorrhagic bone cyst)

2. Aneurysmal bone cyst

---

* These cysts, previously regarded as developmental non-odontogenic cysts, are of debatable origin.

II. CYSTS ASSOCIATED WITH THE MAXILLARY ANTRUM

1. Benign mucosal cyst of the maxillary antrum
2. Surgical ciliated cyst of maxilla

III. CYSTS OF THE SOFT TISSUES OF THE MOUTH, FACE AND NECK

1. Dermoid and epidermoid cysts
2. Branchial cleft (lympho-epithelial) cyst
3. Thyroglossal duct cyst
4. Anterior median lingual cyst
5. Oral cysts with gastric or intestinal epithelium
6. Cysts of the salivary glands
7. Parasitic cysts: hydatid cyst: *Cysticercus cellulosae*

IV. *pseudobranial cysts:*
1. *hronicni apces - granlom*
2. *acuten apces - apsko*
3. *granulocelulozni tu ili celulini epulis*
4. *ostrom ameloblastom*
5. *karcinom*
6. *eozinofili granulom*
7. *(hemangiom ili multipul anginlom*
8. *centralni hemangiom*
9. *specifican oyofonja - TBC, lues. actinomicoze*
10. *osteomijelitis i osteoradio neleroze*
11. *ostali tiporoi cysto*
12. *normalne anatomine sfirhure*

CHAPTER 1

HISTORY

JAW cysts are not lesions confined to modern man. Ruffer (1921) in his studies on the palaeopathology of Egypt has described lesions in the jaws of three mummified specimens which appear to be radicular cysts. The first, from a predynastic era, Naga el Deir (*circa* 4500 B.C.), shows a root remnant in the right second premolar region of the maxilla. A cavity is present in the bone at its apex. In the second specimen, which is thought to be from the same period, the mandibular teeth show marked attrition and there is a cystic area in the bone involving the first permanent molar. The third specimen is from Cleopatra's period, Ras el Tin. An oval opening with smooth borders measuring 12×8 mm is present in the outer wall of the alveolar bone in the premolar region. An aperture artificially made through the external wall of the mandible leads into a smooth-walled cavity, 36×20 mm, in which the roots of the canine, lateral incisor and anterior root of the second molar are exposed.

Salama and Hilmy (1951) reported on two specimens from a collection of skulls excavated at Sakara. All belonged to the period of King Unas of the 5th dynasty (*circa* 2800 B.C.). One is an adult skull showing a large radicular cyst in relation to |234. The teeth in relation to the cyst are missing but sockets are present suggesting that the teeth were lost post mortem. The remaining teeth show marked attrition. The cyst has expanded almost to the midline of the palate. The second specimen shows a large multilocular cyst in the left body of an edentulous mandible. There is expansion of both the inner and outer plates of bone. A skull thought to be from the Hellenistic period has been examined by Dascoulis (1960), who found that it contained a radicular cyst.

Celcus, writing in the early part of the first century A.D., is quoted by Lufkin (1938):

It also happens, that from an ulcer of the gums . . . one may have for a long period a discharge of pus, on account of a broken or rotten tooth, or else on account of a disease of the bone; in this case there often exists a fistula.

Then the latter must be opened, the tooth extracted and if any bony fragment exist, this should be removed; and if there be anything else diseased, this should be scraped away.

1

Lufkin also pointed out that alveolar and perialveolar abscesses are commonly seen in palaeopathological studies particularly in Egyptian mummies.

Pierre Fauchard (1746), having described the dentoalveolar abscess and its treatment, wrote:

I have seen many very considerable tumours which could only have been caused by carious teeth . . . Nothing is more frequent than to see these sort of large tumours, of which the results are insignificant or troublesome according to the exciting causes or the treatment applied to dissipate them and to cure radically when they have formed. I have treated a great number with success.

When incisions in the gums have to be made, for the tumours or to keep them open, sufficient dilation is made with sharp instruments and the incision held open so as not to allow it to close too soon. Not to frighten the patient by the introduction of a fresh cutting instrument, recourse must be had to the use of dossils and tampons of charpie or cotton or to properly made tents covered with wax of some ceriate or convenient plaster which should not be disgusting by its taste or smell . . . A prepared sponge will do as well. But the tents must be gradually reduced in size as the wound heals for if used too long it may be very dangerous as I know from experience, and this happens too often . . .

Sometimes it is necessary to take away, to file and remove some portion not only of the gum but even of the alveolus carious or otherwise to procure sufficient aperture for the discharge of matter and for the introduction of medicaments.

Fauchard's 'Sixth Observation' in Chapter 35 of the same work appears to be a case report of a radicular cyst, although he does not give any specific name to the condition he describes.

On the effect of caries of two roots of a tooth which gave rise to a tumour and abscess on the left side of the lower jaw.

On the 6th December 1723 the wife of M. Brizard Concierge and keeper of furniture of the Hotel de Conti having two roots of a second large molar of the left side of the lower jaw carious for some years, this caused a considerable tumour on the same side. I was called to examine this tumour and to extirpate the two roots which I did in the presence of M. Finot (a) and M. Darmagnac (b). The gap which was left by this enabled me to insert my stiletto into the tumour. By this means I ascertained the depth which extended to the base of the maxillary bone. I knew then that the bone was exposed. I made a sufficient incision in the upper part of the gum to give vent to the matter, and, to prevent the opening of the wound being closed too soon, I dressed this lady with a tent of lint covered over with a little white wax. I renewed this tent night and morning and syringed out the wound every time that I dressed it with a lotion made of two ounces of water of ound wort, barley water with cinnamon, balsam of Fioravanti and honey of roses of each one ounce, the whole mixed together. The fourth day I ceased to use the tents and continued to syringe the wound as formerly until the twenty-fifth day when the patient was perfectly cured.

2

Reflexion

If one deferred at first to draw the carious roots and to open up the abscess sufficiently the lodgement of the matter would have formed a new sinus and made greater progress: when it would not have been perhaps possible to end thus happily the cure of this patient.

John Hunter, writing in about 1780 of diseases of the jaw bones, described a type of lesion which appears to be a cyst.

The second of these diseases in the bone . . . is an accumulation of curdly substance; probably it is coagulable lymph, and may be reckoned among the encysted tumours. The ossific inflammation often goes on here, till the bone acquires great size, but in these the outer ossific accumulation is not in proportion to the absorption, and therefore, being only a thin shell, it gives way.

Early work on the nature and treatment of jaw cysts appears in the English literature in papers by Spence (1853–54), Harvey (1855), Moon (1877–78), Heath (1880, 1887) and Pedley (1886).

CHAPTER 2

PRIMORDIAL CYST (KERATOCYST)

[handwritten annotation]

THERE has been a great deal of interest in the primordial cyst since it became apparent that it may grow to a large size before it manifests clinically and that, unlike other jaw cysts, it has a particular tendency to recur following surgical treatment.

The term 'odontogenic keratocyst' was introduced by Philipsen (1956) and is now very widely used. In this and in a subsequent paper (Pindborg, Philipsen and Henriksen, 1962), and in a paper by Pindborg and Hansen (1963), the designation 'keratocyst' was used to describe any jaw cyst in which keratin was formed to a large extent. Some follicular, radicular and residual cysts were therefore included in the category of odontogenic keratocyst.

Although a few radicular and residual cyst linings may become keratinized by metaplasia (*Fig.* 1), these linings are distinctly different from the characteristic lining epithelium of the primordial cyst (Browne, 1971a). While primordial cyst linings do keratinize, they have other features which distinguish them and it is these which are probably responsible for their biological behaviour, rather than the presence of keratin. Lucas (1972) has made the point that the emphasis that has been placed on keratinization is to some extent misleading, in that there is the implication that cysts of widely differing types may all keratinize and that if they do they are then liable to recur. There is now a great deal of evidence that the cyst under discussion here is a distinct entity of developmental origin, arising from primordial odontogenic epithelium, and it is for this reason that I prefer the term 'primordial cyst' to the non-specific histological term 'keratocyst'.

Browne (1969, 1972) has shown that keratinizing cysts have a significantly ($P < 1$ per cent) different age distribution (mean age 32·1 yr; peak in second and third decades) from dentigerous (mean age 36·6 yr; peak in fifth decade) and radicular cysts (mean age 40·2 yr; peak from third to sixth decades). He concluded from this that the three types of cyst arise from different populations and that the keratocyst is therefore a distinct lesion in its own right. The fact that it occurs at a younger age than the others makes it unlikely that it has arisen in long-standing dentigerous or radicular cysts.

Browne (1969), and Hjørting-Hansen et al. (1969) have demonstrated, moreover, that the site distribution of keratinizing cysts differs significantly ($P < 1$ per cent) from that of non-keratinized cysts;

4

a fact which has been confirmed by Rud and Pindborg (1969) who believed that this supported the assumption that keratocysts are actually primordial cysts. Hjørting-Hansen and co-workers found no evidence to suggest that a primary unkeratinized odontogenic cyst has become keratinized.

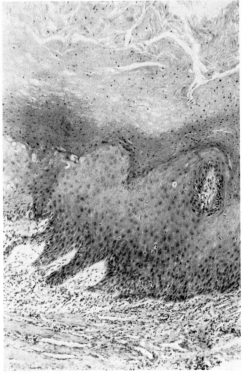

Fig. 1. Parakeratinized stratified squamous epithelium lining a radicular cyst. HE; × 75.

Despite agreeing that these cysts are distinct entities, Browne (1969) argued that they cannot be primordial cysts because he defines a primordial cyst as one which arises by breakdown of the stellate reticulum of the enamel organ before any mineralized tissue is formed and hence develops in place of a tooth which may be one of the normal series or a supernumerary. If, however, one defines a primordial cyst as one which arises from primordial odontogenic epithelium, i.e. dental lamina or its remnants (Soskolne and Shear, 1967; Toller, 1967), or enamel organ prior to tooth formation, this would seem to define more accurately the possible histogenesis of this cyst and to distinguish it from other jaw cysts in which the epithelial linings have keratinized by metaplasia.

5

Clinical Features

Frequency

Our own material comprises 84 primordial cysts (11·2 per cent) of a total of 750 cysts of the jaws accessioned over a 15-year period (*Table* 1). The 84 cysts occurred in 69 patients. The frequency in other studies is shown in *Table* 2.

Table 1.
DISTRIBUTION OF 750 JAW CYSTS ACCORDING TO DIAGNOSIS

Cyst	Number	Percentage
Radicular/residual	433	57·7
Dentigerous	103	13·7
Nasopalatine	89	11·9
Primordial	84	11·2
'Globulomaxillary'	17	2·3
Solitary	8	1·1
Eruption	7	0·9
Nasolabial	5	0·7
Lateral periodontal	2	0·3
Gingival	1	0·1
Aneurysmal	1	0·1
Total	750	100

Table 2.
FREQUENCY OF PRIMORDIAL CYSTS IN DIFFERENT SERIES

Author(s)	Material	Percentage Primordial
Pindborg et al., 1962	26 of 791 odontogenic	3.3
Toller, 1967	33 of 300 cysts of all types	11·0
Browne, 1970	41 of 537 odontogenic cysts	7·6
Main, 1970a	12 of 289 epithelial jaw cysts	4·2
Stoelinga, 1971	54 of 486 jaw cysts	11·1
Killey and Kay, 1972	25 of 746 jaw cysts	3·3
Payne, 1972	103 of 1313 odontogenic	7·8
Radden and Reade, 1973	64 of 368 odontogenic	17·4
Shear, present study	{ 84 of 750 jaw cysts	11·2
	{ 84 of 647 odontogenic	13·0

Age

A number of series have now been published. Primordial cysts occur over a wide age range and cases have been recorded as early as the first decade and as late as the ninth. In most series there has been a pronounced peak incidence in the second and third decades, with figures ranging from 48 per cent to 60 per cent of patients being in this age group. The ages at diagnosis of 61 primordial cysts from our own material are shown in *Fig.* 2.

6

Sex

Primordial cysts are generally found more frequently in males than in females ($P < 5$ per cent) and although this sex predilection appears to be more marked in Black than in White patients, the difference is not statistically significant ($P > 10$ per cent). In a series of 67 of

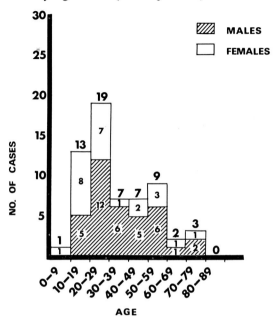

Fig. 2. Ages of patients at diagnosis of 61 primordial cysts.

our patients, there were approximately twice as many males as females. Of these, 33 were White males and 21 White females (1·6 : 1); 11 were Black males and 2 Black females (5·5 : 1) (*Table* 3).

Table 3.
SEX DISTRIBUTION OF BLACK AND WHITE PATIENTS WITH PRIMORDIAL CYSTS

	Male	Female	Total	M : F Ratio
Black	11	2	13	5·5 : 1
White	33	21	54	1·6 : 1
Total	44 (66%)	23 (34%)	67	1·9 : 1
W : B ratio	3 : 1	10·5 : 1	4·2 : 1	

The preponderance of White patients involved is also noteworthy as the White : Black population ratio on the Witwatersrand, from which most of our material is drawn, is 1 : 1·6.

7

Site

The mandible is involved far more frequently than the maxilla. In our own material, 51 of 69 cysts (74 per cent) have occurred in the mandible. Browne (1970) recorded an 83 per cent incidence in the mandible and Pindborg and Hansen (1963) and Hansen (1967) a 77 per cent incidence. About one-half of all primordial cysts occur at the angle of the mandible extending for varying distances into the ascending ramus and forward into the body. As to the site distribution of the other cases, reports of a number of studies indicate that they can occur anywhere in the jaws including the midline of the mandible and maxilla and the 'globulomaxillary area' in the maxilla.

Clinical Presentation

Patients with primordial cysts complain of either pain, swelling or discharge. Some of our patients have been unaware of the lesions until they developed pathological fractures. Some of these cysts have been discovered fortuitously during dental examination when radiographs were taken. In many instances, patients are remarkably free of symptoms until the cysts have reached a large size, involving the entire ascending ramus. This is because the primordial cyst tends to extend in the medullary cavity and expansion of the bone occurs late. As with many other intraosseous jaw lesions, the enlarging cyst may produce displacement of the teeth.

An analysis of the location and incidence of bony expansion has been made by Browne (1970). In his study, expansion of bone occurred in about 60 per cent of cases. One-third of maxillary cysts caused buccal expansion, but palatal expansion was very rarely seen. About a half of the mandibular lesions produced buccal expansion and one-third produced lingual expansion. The great majority of the latter group were in the third molar or ascending ramus regions.

Multiple primordial cysts are found in some patients. Of 69 patients in our series, 62 had single cysts and 7 (10 per cent) had more than one. In 3 of the latter, the cysts were part of the naevoid basal cell carcinoma syndrome. Of these patients, one has had 6 cysts, another 5 and one has had 2.

Recurrences

Brief reference has already been made to the fact that the primordial cyst has a particular tendency to recur after surgical treatment. The recurrences in various reported series is shown in *Table* 4. Pindborg and Hansen (1963) were the first to point out this peculiarly aggressive behaviour. They reported a recurrence rate of 62 per cent in a series of 16 cysts and observed that there was no correlation between the size or location of the cyst and its tendency to recur; nor was there any difference in recurrence rate between cases which were treated by

8

'extirpation' and those treated by 'fenestration'. Hansen (1967) found a recurrence rate of 52 per cent in a series of 52 cases followed for a period of at least 6 months. Browne (1970) reported a 25 per cent recurrence rate in 85 cysts followed for 6 months or longer.

Table 4.
RECURRENCES OF PRIMORDIAL CYSTS IN VARIOUS SERIES

Author(s)	Number of cases followed	Recurrence rate per cent
Pindborg and Hansen, 1963	16	62
Hansen, 1967	52	52
Toller, 1967	55	51
Rud and Pindborg, 1969	21	33
Panders and Hadders, 1969	22	14
Browne, 1970	85	25
Stoelinga, 1971	54	10
Payne, 1972	20	45
Butz, 1975	38	11
Eversole et al., 1975	35	20

He found that most recurrences occurred in the first 5 years after surgery but one of his cases recurred 20 years after operation. Bramley (1971) reported a case with a recurrence 40 years after surgical treatment. Browne (1970) could find no statistically significant correlation between the frequency of recurrence and the age of the patient, location of the cyst, the method of treatment (enucleation or marsupialization), the nature of the cyst lining, and the presence of cortical perforation. In a later paper Browne (1971a) showed that there was a very similar rate of recurrence following removal of cysts with satellite cysts (23·7 per cent) and those without satellite cysts (24·4 per cent). There was a higher frequency of recurrence of cysts without epithelial residues (28·1 per cent) than with (8·3 per cent) but the difference was not statistically significant.

The recurrence rate in Toller's material (1967) was 51 per cent of 55 cysts and Rud and Pindborg (1969) reported a recurrence rate of 33 per cent of 21 cysts. Toller (1971) summarized the findings of a number of different groups of workers. In a total of 195 patients there were 85 first recurrences (44 per cent). In our own sample, 38 patients have been followed-up from between 8 months and 17 years. There are 2 definite recurrences, proved at operation and histologically, and a further 2 probable cases on the basis of radiological evidence are being carefully watched (Butz, 1975). This constitutes a recurrence rate of 11 per cent. Of the definite recurrences, one was discovered 2½ years and the other 1 year after the original operation. Lower recurrence rates than in most other studies have also been reported by Panders and Hadders in 1969 (14 per cent) and by Stoelinga in 1971 (10 per cent).

9

There are a number of possible reasons why primordial cysts recur so frequently. The first of these is related to their tendency to multiplicity in some patients, including the occurrence of satellite cysts which are retained during an enucleation procedure. Some instances of recurrence are likely therefore to be new cysts rather than true recurrences. Secondly, primordial cyst linings are very thin and fragile, particularly when the cysts are large, and are therefore more difficult to enucleate than cysts with thick walls. Portions of the lining may be left behind (Kramer, 1963; Fickling, 1965) and constitute the origin of a recurrence. Toller (1967) has suggested in this context that the epithelial linings of primordial cysts have intrinsic growth potential and believes that there is some reason for regarding them as benign neoplasms. Another possibility is suggested by evidence derived from patients with the naevoid basal cell carcinoma syndrome. These patients have a particular predisposition to form primordial cysts from the dental lamina (Soskolne and Shear, 1967). This suggests that primordial cysts in patients without the syndrome may also possibly arise from the dental lamina. If these individuals also have an inherent tendency to develop such cysts, then any remnants of dental lamina may form the target for primordial cyst formation.

Payne (1972) compared the histological features of recurrent primordial cysts with non-recurrent specimens and those from patients with the naevoid basal cell carcinoma syndrome. The presence of inflammation and the type of keratin produced did not seem to be significant. He found bud-like proliferations of the basal cell layer in 5 of 11 recurrent cysts (45 per cent) and 4 of 9 cysts from patients with the syndrome (44 per cent). By comparison, only 6 of 72 non-recurrent primordial cysts (8 per cent) showed this feature. Satellite microcysts were observed in the cyst walls of 78 per cent of cysts from patients with the syndrome, 18 per cent of the recurrent cysts and 4 per cent of the non-recurrent cysts.

Yet another possible source of the recurrences has been suggested by Stoelinga (1971) and Stoelinga and Peters (1973) who have proposed that the cysts may arise from proliferations of the basal cells of the oral mucosa particularly in the third molar region and ascending ramus of the mandible. They referred to the fact that there is often firm adhesion of the cysts to the overlying mucosa and recommended that when they are surgically removed, the overlying mucosa should be excised with them in an attempt to prevent possible recurrence from residual basal cell proliferations.

As oral surgeons have become increasingly aware of the need to treat primordial cysts more aggressively than other jaw cysts, it is likely that future studies will show a declining incidence of recurrences.

Enlargement

Reference has already been made to Toller's view that primordial cysts might possibly be regarded as benign neoplasms. There is not much information about their rate of growth. As they tend to extend along the cancellous component of the bone without producing much expansion of the cortical plates, they frequently reach a large size, particularly at the angle of mandible and ascending ramus, before they are diagnosed. Although Browne (1971a) was of the opinion that these cysts grow more rapidly than other jaw cysts, Toller's view (1967) was that they grow at a similar rate to other epithelial cysts of the jaws. He suggested that the majority of primordial cysts would take about 6 years to recur to a clinically significant size of more than 1 cm diameter but the range of growth rates in his experience varied from 1 to 25 years. The significant point appears to be, as put by Main (1970b), that although the rate of enlargement of primordial cysts may not be greater than that of other jaw cysts, its growth is more unremitting. The reason for this unremitting growth has been investigated by both Main (1970a) and Toller (1971). Main showed that the mitotic value of primordial cyst epithelial linings ranged from 0 to 19 with a mean of 8·0. This figure was similar to that in the ameloblastoma and in dental lamina, and higher than that found in non-odontogenic cysts which had a mean mitotic value of 2·3, and radicular cysts with a mean mitotic value of 4·5.

Toller estimated mitotic activity by autoradiography following the *in vitro* incubation of cyst linings in tissue culture medium to which had been added tritiated thymidine. The mean labelling indices were 13·0 per cent for a series of 6 primordial cysts compared with 1·7 per cent for 5 non-primordial jaw cysts. The mean figure for human buccal mucous membrane was 7·0 per cent.

Toller (1970b) also considered the role played by the osmolality of the cyst fluid in enlargement of the primordial cysts. He showed that there was a mean osmolality of $296 \pm 15·6$ milliosmoles (11 cases) compared with a serum osmolality of $282 \pm 14·75$ milliosmoles. This difference is statistically significant at the 1 per cent level. In view of the low total soluble protein level in primordial cysts (Toller, 1970a), he suggested that osmotic differences between sera and cyst fluids are not directly related to proteins in cyst fluids and may be the result of the liberation of the products of cell lysis which may not be proteins. He believed strongly that the raised osmolalities play an important, even if not the sole, role in the expansive growth in the size of the primordial as well as other jaw cysts.

Main (1970b) on the other hand, felt that mural growth in the form of epithelial proliferation is the essential process involved in the enlargement of primordial cysts and that the evidence for osmotic diffusion is inconclusive.

11

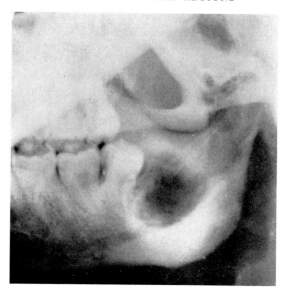

Fig. 3. Radiograph of unilocular primordial cyst posterior to mandibular third molar tooth. It is unilocular and has a smooth periphery.

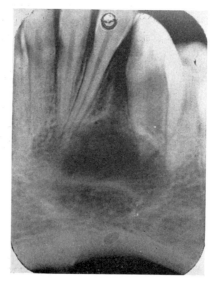

Fig. 4. Radiograph of unilocular primordial cyst in anterior region of mandible. The cyst has a smooth periphery.

12

Donoff et al. (1972) have demonstrated the presence of collageno-lytic activity on skin collagen in explant and tissue cultures of primordial cysts but only when both epithelium and fibrous wall were present in the media. No similar activity was demonstrable in dentigerous cysts. They tentatively proposed that enzymatic mechanisms may be important in the growth of primordial cysts.

Radiological Features

Primordial cysts may appear radiologically as small round or ovoid radiolucent areas. Frequently however the lesions are more extensive. Most of them are well-demarcated with a distinct sclerotic margin as might be expected from a slowly-enlarging lesion. The majority are unilocular radiolucencies, and most of these have a smooth periphery (*Figs.* 3 and 4). Almost all the maxillary lesions are of this variety and tend to be small as they make their clinical appearance earlier than the mandibular lesions. Some of the unilocular lesions have scalloped margins (*Fig.* 5) and these may be

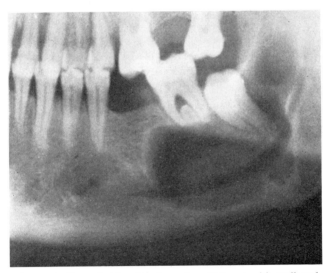

Fig. 5. Radiograph of unilocular primordial cyst with scalloped margins.

misinterpreted as multilocular lesions. The scalloped margins suggest that unequal growth activity may be taking place in different parts of the cyst lining. True multilocular lesions are not un-common, and Browne (1970) found 19 of 83 cysts (30 per cent) to be of this type, all in the mandible. This variety is particularly liable

13

to be diagnosed as ameloblastoma (*Fig. 6*). There may be extensive involvement of the body and ascending ramus of the mandible, with little or no bony expansion.

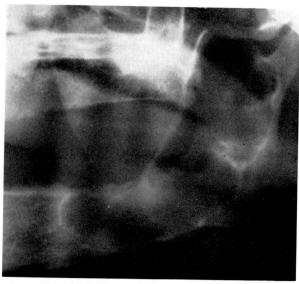

Fig. 6. Radiograph of a multilocular primordial cyst. The multi-locularity was confirmed at operation. (*Courtesy of Dr. J. Lownie.*)

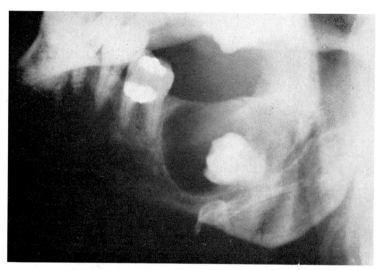

Fig. 7. Radiograph of primordial cyst which has enveloped an unerupted tooth to produce a 'dentigerous' appearance.

14

Primordial cysts may impede the eruption of related teeth and this results in a 'dentigerous' appearance radiologically (*Fig. 7*). These lesions are frequently misdiagnosed as dentigerous cysts and this has given rise to two misconceptions (*Fig. 8*). One is that many dentigerous cysts have keratinized epithelial linings similar to those found in primordial cysts; and the second is that dentigerous cysts may have an extrafollicular origin (Gillette and Weinmann, 1958).

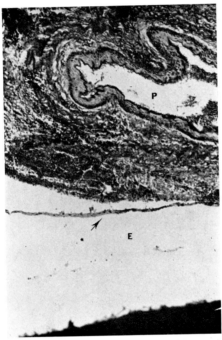

Fig. 8. Primordial cyst (**P**) which has enveloped an unerupted tooth. Enamel space (**E**). Reduced enamel epithelium of unerupted tooth indicated with an arrow. Picromallory; ×50.

For all this, the point should be made that, very occasionally, the lining of a true dentigerous cyst may be identical to that of a primordial cyst. It has been suggested (Browne, 1969) that this occurs when an enlarging primordial cyst involves the follicle of an unerupted tooth and fuses with the reduced enamel epithelium. He pointed out that in such cysts the epithelium immediately around the neck of the tooth is not keratinized and shows inflammatory changes in the underlying capsule. Main (1970a) has referred to the variety of primordial cyst which embraces an adjacent unerupted tooth as 'envelopmental'. Those cysts which form in the place of a

15

normal tooth of the series, he called the 'replacement' variety; those in the ascending ramus away from the teeth he referred to as 'extraneous'. Main proposed the use of the term 'collateral' for those primordial cysts adjacent to the roots of teeth, usually in the mandibular premolar region, which are indistinguishable radiologically from the lateral periodontal cyst (*Fig. 9*, and *Fig.* 24 (p. 36)).

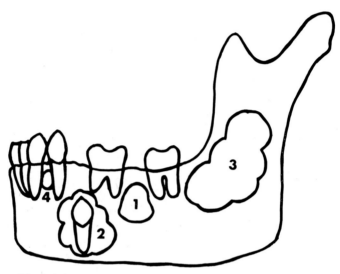

Fig. 9. Diagram illustrating the varieties of primordial cyst, drawn after Main (1970a). 1. Replacement; 2. Envelopmental; 3. Extraneous; 4. Collateral.

Primordial cysts may, as they enlarge, produce deflection of roots of teeth, but only very rarely do they appear to cause root resorption (Struthers and Shear, 1976).

Finally, primordial cysts may present radiologically in the globulomaxillary and median mandibular regions. The question as to whether globulomaxillary and median mandibular cysts in fact exist is controversial and is discussed in Chapter 9.

Pathogenesis

Most of the available evidence suggests that the primordial cyst arises from odontogenic epithelium prior to tooth formation; in other words, the dental lamina or its remnants, and possibly the enamel organ before tooth formation commences. It was originally believed that all primordial cysts were derived from an enamel organ, either of the normal dentition, in which case a tooth would be

16

missing, or from a supernumerary bud. There is still no evidence to indicate that the possibility of such an origin must be entirely excluded. It is possible, although by no means certain, that the 'replacement' variety described by Main may develop from an enamel organ of the normal tooth series. It is also possible however that a 'replacement' cyst might arise from a portion of the dental lamina which was destined to become an enamel organ (the so-called tooth primordium) and that the enamel organ subsequently fails to differentiate.

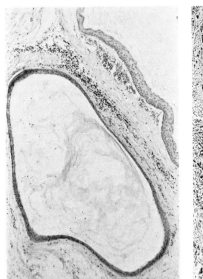 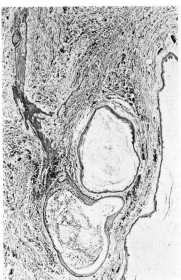

Fig. 10. Fig. 11.

Fig. 10. Satellite microcyst in the wall of a primordial cyst. HE; ×50.

Fig. 11. Satellite microcysts in the wall of a primordial cyst, apparently arising directly from the dental lamina in a patient with the naevoid basal cell carcinoma syndrome. HE; ×20.

As mentioned earlier, evidence derived mainly from the examination of primordial cysts from patients with the naevoid basal cell carcinoma syndrome suggests that the cysts may arise directly from dental lamina (Soskolne and Shear, 1967). Satellite microcysts in the walls of the main cysts are often seen apparently arising directly from remnants of the dental lamina (*Figs.* 10 and 11). The stimulus for this phenomenon is not known, but as the naevoid basal cell carcinoma syndrome is transmitted genetically as an autosomal dominant (Gorlin and Goltz, 1960), and the occurrence of multiple

17

primordial cysts in patients with the syndrome is a common finding, it is possible that there is a predisposition in some individuals to form primordial cysts and it may be for this reason that they are so frequently multiple. Browne (1969) suggested that as the naevoid basal cell carcinoma syndrome can appear in varying degrees of completeness, the presence of a cyst without other features of the syndrome may represent the least complete form. No one has yet

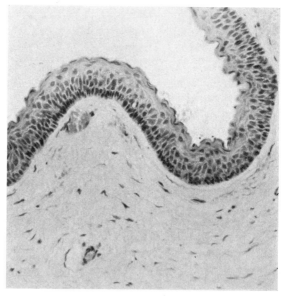

Fig. 12. Primordial cyst. HE; ×185.

demonstrated a familial tendency to develop primordial cysts in the absence of other features of the syndrome, and although the possibility that their occurrence may be genetically determined cannot be excluded, it must be regarded at present as speculation.

The epithelial linings of some satellite cysts appear to degenerate, but in others continue to proliferate and establish multilocular lesions (Browne, 1969).

Stoelinga (1971, 1973) has proposed a third possible origin of primordial cysts. He suggested that they may arise from proliferations of basal cells of the oral mucosa, forming what he termed 'basal cell hamartias'.

The consistent finding of a keratinized layer in primordial cysts, while this feature is so rarely seen in other jaw cysts, may be related to their origin from dental lamina. It has often been noted that dental lamina can give rise to keratin (Hjørting-Hansen et al., 1969).

18

orotinised stratified squamous epithelium

Dentigerous cysts are lined by reduced enamel epithelium which usually does not appear to have the capacity for keratinization, and radicular cysts develop from cell rests of Malassez which likewise seem to have very little potential for keratinization. Bartlett et al. (1973) have shown that keratinizing cysts form in the enamel organ epithelium of tooth germs transplanted in the kidneys of isologous mice and this provides a potentially useful experimental model for the investigation of primordial cysts.

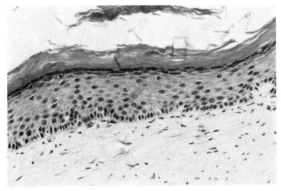

Fig. 13. Primordial cyst lined by orthokeratinized stratified squamous epithelium. HE; × 185.

Pathology

Unless the cyst is very small, the linings of primordial cysts are rarely received intact in the laboratory. They are invariably thin-walled, collapsed and folded.

The histological features are characteristic (Shear, 1960a). The cysts are lined by a regular keratinized stratified squamous epithelium which is usually about 5–8 cell layers thick and without rete ridges (*Fig. 12*). The form of keratinization is predominantly parakeratotic but is sometimes orthokeratotic (*Fig. 13*) and both forms are found in different parts of some cysts. A stratum granulosum is associated with the orthokeratin layer in some but not all cases. The parakeratotic layers often have a corrugated surface. There is a well-defined basal layer consisting usually of columnar cells and occasionally cuboidal cells. The nuclei frequently tend to be orientated away from the basement membrane and in the majority of cases are intensely basophilic. Desquamated keratin is present in many of the cyst cavities. The cells superficial to the basal layer are polyhedral and often have intracellular oedema. Mitotic figures are found in the basal layer but more frequently in the suprabasal layers (Browne,

19

1971a). Some linings (*Figs.* 14*a*, *b*, 15 and 16) show features of epithelial dysplasia (Rud and Pindborg, 1969) and some workers, while stressing that malignant transformation in jaw cysts is extremely rare, make the point that keratinizing cysts appear to have a greater tendency to such change than others (Toller, 1967). Browne and Gough (1972), proposed that keratin metaplasia in an

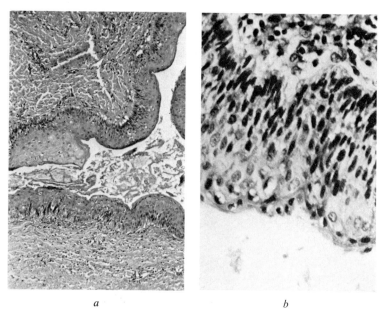

a   b

Fig. 14*a*, Primordial cyst lining with epithelial dysplasia. HE; ×60.
b, A different area of the cyst illustrated in *Fig.* 14*a*, showing the epithelial dysplasia. HE; ×310.

otherwise non-keratinized odontogenic cyst may indicate carcinomatous potential. They indicated however that there is little evidence that the primordial cyst is associated with malignant change more commonly than other types of odontogenic cyst.

Vedtofte and Dabelsteen (1975) have studied the expression of blood group antigens A and B in 8 ameloblastomas, 16 primordial cysts from patients with the naevoid basal cell carcinoma syndrome, 11 primordial cysts from patients without the syndrome, and 12 non-keratinizing odontogenic cysts, using a double layer immunofluorescence staining technique. All ameloblastomas reacted negatively, 3 cysts from the patients with the naevoid basal cell carcinoma syndrome reacted negatively and the primordial cysts from patients without the syndrome, as well as the non-keratinizing

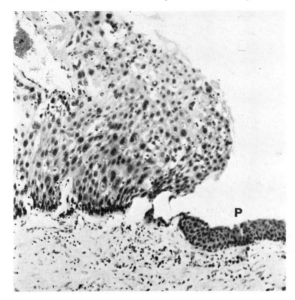

Fig. 15. Primordial cyst lining (P) showing severe epithelial dysplasia. (*Section lent by Professor J. J. Pindborg.*) HE; ×90.

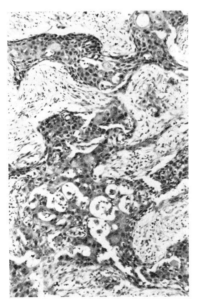

Fig. 16. Infiltrating squamous carcinoma in another area of the cyst illustrated in *Fig.* 15. HE; ×60.

odontogenic cysts, all gave a positive reaction. This is of interest in view of other studies (Dabelsteen and Fulling, 1971) which showed that there was a loss of blood group antigens A and B in dysplastic epithelium compared with normal oral epithelium.

The fibrous capsule of the primordial cyst is usually thin with relatively few cells widely separated by a stroma which is often rich in mucopolysaccharide and resembles mesenchymal connective tissue (*Fig.* 12). Inflammatory cells are very infrequent but there

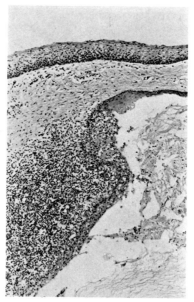

Fig. 17. Inflamed portion of the wall of a primordial cyst. HE; ×50.

may be a mild infiltration of lymphocytes and monocytes. In the presence of an intense inflammatory process, the adjacent epithelium loses its keratinized surface, may thicken and develop rete processes or may ulcerate (*Fig.* 17). Hyalinization is sometimes seen in the capsules of cysts removed from older patients (Browne, 1971a).

The attachment between epithelium and fibrous wall tends to be weak and in many areas they separate. The collapsed and folded thin-walled cysts may give an erroneous impression of multi-locularity in histological sections.

Satellite cysts and proliferating dental lamina are sometimes seen in the cyst capsules, particularly in patients with the naevoid basal cell carcinoma syndrome (*Fig.* 11). Although the epithelial linings of the cysts in the syndrome patients usually show the classic features of primordial cysts, Waldron (1969) has described some histologic variants. In some of his syndrome cases the epithelial linings were considerably thicker than in classic cases and showed prominent nests of basaloid cells budding off from the cyst linings. Mucous metaplasia, hyaline bodies (Rushton, 1955) and cholesterol clefts are occasionally present in the walls of primordial cysts (Browne, 1971a) and an ultrastructural study of a series of them has been reported by Hansen and Kobayasi (1970b).

Estimation of the soluble protein level in aspirated cyst fluid may be a valuable aid in the preoperative diagnosis of primordial cysts. Toller (1970a) has shown that fluids from keratinizing cysts have soluble protein levels below 3·5 g per 100 ml (mean 2·2 g per 100 ml), whereas the values for non-keratinizing cysts were in the range 5·0–11·0 g per 100 ml with a mean of 7·1 g per 100 ml. Electrophoretic studies corroborated the finding that keratinizing cysts are very low in soluble proteins and Toller felt that a protein level of less than 4·0 g per 100 ml indicated a diagnosis of primordial cyst. A value of over 5·0 g per 100 ml, however, would suggest a radicular, dentigerous or fissural cyst, or even an ameloblastoma. He postulated that fully keratinized linings are impervious to all proteins whereas the usual type of radicular or dentigerous cyst wall will at least slowly transmit the smaller proteins. In the presence of a fairly pronounced inflammatory reaction in a primordial cyst wall, the degree of keratinization over these areas will be altered and this is likely to increase the permeability of the lining and result in a soluble protein level in the fluid higher than in the uninflamed keratinizing cysts.

Kramer suggested in 1970 that a preoperative diagnosis of primordial cyst might be made by aspirating cyst fluid and demonstrating keratinized squames in a stained film. In a later study, Kramer and Toller (1973) reported on the combined use of exfoliative cytology and protein estimations in the preoperative diagnosis of these cysts. In some instances, when aspirates were sent in the post, a period of up to two days had elapsed before smears were prepared, but whenever practicable smears should be done as soon as possible after sampling. Smears are made by placing a drop of fluid on a clean glass slide and spreading with the edge of a dry coverslip. Two smears of each specimen are allowed to air-dry and are stained respectively with haematoxylin–eosin and by the Rhodamine B fluorescence method (Clausen and Dabelsteen, 1969). A third is allowed to dry to a tacky state and fixed in a solution containing 75 per cent ethyl alcohol and 3 per cent acetic acid prior to staining with the Papanicolaou procedure.

Kramer and Toller examined a total of 56 jaw cysts and of these subsequent histological examination showed that 21 were primordial cysts, 32 were simple cysts and 3 were cystic neoplasms.

23

Examination for squames gave the correct result, namely primordial cyst or not primordial cyst, in 47 of the 56 cases. When this cytological procedure was combined with protein estimation of cyst fluid, the correct diagnosis was reached in all 21 primordial cysts. There were 6 false positives among the other cysts and squames were also found in the fluid from a cystic carcinoma.

They found that examination of the exfoliative cytology smears achieves comparable diagnostic accuracy with each of the three staining methods and that this accuracy was similar to that achieved by use of the protein estimations. Although none of the methods gives complete accuracy, the number of incorrect diagnoses is reduced if smears stained by two or three methods and protein estimations are performed on each case. The smear technique requires very little material and this can almost always be aspirated even if the cyst contents are thick.

As it is so important from the point of view of treatment of primordial cysts that a correct preoperative diagnosis be established, these diagnostic procedures can be of considerable value.

Toller and Holborow (1969) examined 15 jaw cyst fluids by immuno-electrophoresis and found that cysts with keratinized epithelial linings had the lowest levels of immunoglobulins.

Treatment

In view of the now well-known tendency for the primordial cyst to recur, its treatment has given rise to much discussion among oral surgeons. There have been reports of success and failure with both enucleation and marsupialization procedures. It has been suggested that an explanation for those marsupialization procedures which have been successful may be that the proliferative potential of primordial cyst lining only manifests in the cystic situation. Marsupialization, it has been suggested, will only be successful provided that no satellite cysts are left behind.

My own opinion is that the treatment of primordial cysts by marsupialization is incorrect in principle in view of the evidence that proliferating dental lamina and developing satellite cysts may occur in the fibrous wall of the primary cyst cavity.

Bramley (1971, 1974) has suggested what appears to be a rational approach to the treatment of these cysts. He emphasized that serious attempts must be applied to achieve definitive treatment at the first operation. This depends on excellent surgical access, and underestimation of the difficulties of surgical accessibility at the first operation frequently leads to failure. Small single lesions with regular spherical outline can usually be completely enucleated provided access is good. For cysts close to the surface, the overlying mucoperiosteum should be excised at the same time.

24

Larger or less accessible cysts should be carefully enucleated by an extraoral approach if an intraoral approach would result in blind curettage. Great care must be taken during every enucleation procedure to ensure that all fragments of the extremely thin lining are removed. The unilocular lesions with scalloped margins cause much more difficulty. Bramley recommended that these, and the small multilocular lesion, should be treated by marginal excision, with overlying mucosa. If there are any difficulties of access, extraoral exposure is necessary.

For the large multilocular lesions, excision and immediate bone-graft is the treatment of choice at the first operation. If the lesion is deemed to have perforated the bone then an extraperiosteal excision is indicated, together with excision of overlying muscle covering the presumed area of penetration.

Primordial cysts can involve the related soft tissues. Emerson et al. (1972) reported two such examples and warned that in treating these cases the oral surgeon should take care to avoid contamination of the tissues by cyst epithelium.

Clearly, every cyst and every patient should be assessed individually and the treatment planned carefully for each case. Whatever form of surgical approach is selected, the patient should be reviewed regularly. Toller (1972) suggested that re-examination of patients, including radiography, should be done after 6 months, 1 year, 3 years and 7 years.

CHAPTER 3

GINGIVAL CYST OF INFANTS

Clinical Features

THE frequency of gingival cysts is high in newborn infants but they are rarely seen after 3 months of age. It is apparent that most of them undergo involution and disappear, or rupture through the surface epithelium and exfoliate, as very few are submitted for

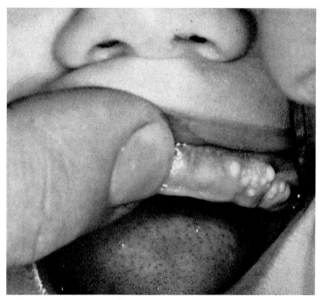

Fig. 18. Gingival cysts in an infant. (*Courtesy of Professor J. J. Pindborg.*)

pathological examination. Monteleone and McLellan (1964) and Fromm (1967) have done extensive clinical surveys of newborn infants to look for nodules in the mouth, frequently referred to as Bohn's nodules or Epstein's pearls. There is some confusion about the two eponyms and their relation to gingival cysts. It would appear that Epstein's pearls are those which occur along the mid-palatine raphe and are not of odontogenic origin, whereas Bohn's nodules are found on the buccal or lingual aspects of the dental ridges. Fromm (1967) pointed out moreover that Bohn was writing about remnants of mucous glands and Bohn had called them 'mucous gland cysts'. Gingival cysts, according to Fromm, are found only on the crests of the maxillary and mandibular dental ridges. For all this, the three terms are frequently used synonymously.

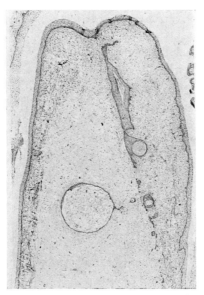

Fig. 19. Fragmentation of dental lamina with formation of microcysts containing keratin in the developing alveolus of a human embryo C. R. 135 mm. (*Section lent by Professor C. W. van Wyk*.) Van Gieson; ×20.

Monteleone and McLellan found nodules in the midpalatine raphe region of 79 per cent of Negro infants and 85 per cent of Caucasian infants. The incidence in Fromm's study was 76 per cent, most of which were along the midpalatal raphe at the junction of hard and soft palates. They were found less frequently along the maxillary dental ridge and least of all along the crest of the mandibular ridge. The nodules were 2–3 mm in diameter. Some infants had only one cyst, some had many, but usually there were five or six. Very few infants had more than one or two along the dental ridges. They are white or cream-coloured (*Fig. 18*). Their absence from the soft palate was explained by Burdi (1968) whose embryologic studies suggested that a consolidation of the soft palate and uvula takes place not by fusion but by subepithelial mesenchymal merging of bilateral primordia without direct apposition and breakdown of epithelium.

27

Common as they are in infants, gingival cysts are extremely rare over 3 months of age. Saunders (1972) however has reported a case in a 3-month-old child and some occur in adults although these are of a different nature and are discussed in Chapter 4.

Pathogenesis

There is general agreement that gingival cysts in infants arise from the dental lamina. Stout et al. (1968) studied epithelial remnants in fetal, infant and adult material. In human fetuses aged between

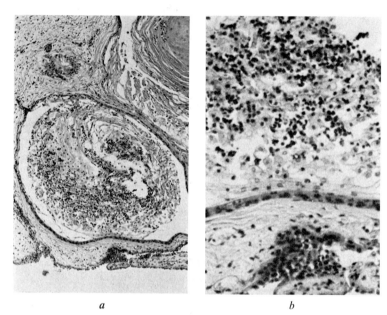

a   b

Fig. 20*a*, Gingival cyst in an infant. (*Section lent by Professor W. G. Shafer.*) HE; ×50. *b*, Higher magnification of portion of the gingival cyst illustrated in *Fig.* 20*a*. HE; ×150.

10 and 12 weeks there was evidence of small amounts of keratin formation in fragmented portions of dental lamina. By late in the twelfth week the dental laminae were fragmented and many fragments showed keratin cyst formation (*Fig.* 19). They found epithelial remnants or gingival cysts in the maxillae of 109 infants ranging in age from birth to 4 years who were examined at autopsy. In their adult material, only 1 of 266 subjects had a cyst although epithelial rests were demonstrated in 90.

The epithelial remnants of the dental lamina have the capacity, at an early stage in development, to proliferate, keratinize and form small cysts. This ability to proliferate is of limited potential, unlike that of the dental lamina in the formation and growth of primordial cysts. Some of the gingival cysts probably open on to the surface leaving clefts; others may be involved by developing teeth. Some degenerate and disappear, the keratin and debris being digested by giant cells. Saunders (1972) reported that when he incised the epithelium over one of these cysts the contents were ejected, suggesting that they might be under pressure. Very few, as previously mentioned, become clinical problems.

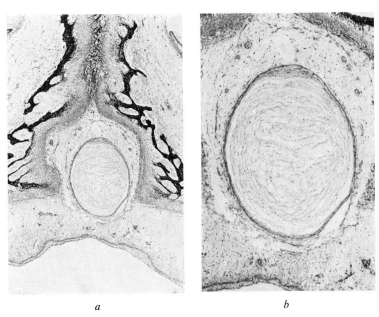

a   b

Fig. 21a, Midpalatal raphe cyst in a human embryo C.R. 135 mm. (*Section lent by Professor C. W. van Wyk.*) Van Gieson; ×20. b, Higher magnification of midpalatal raphe cyst illustrated in *Fig. 21a.* HE; ×45.

The cysts along the midpalatal raphe have a different origin. They arise from epithelial inclusions at the line of fusion of the palatal folds and the nasal processes. This is normally completed by the end of the fourth month. After birth the epithelial inclusions usually atrophy and become resorbed. Some may however produce keratin-containing microcysts (*Figs.* 21a, b) which extend to the surface and rupture during the first few months after birth. Burke et al. (1966) confirmed the presence of frequent palatine raphe cysts but suggested the possibility that they may represent abortive glandular differentiation leading to cyst formation.

Pathology

The cysts are round or ovoid and may have a smooth or an undulating outline in histological sections. There is a thin lining of stratified squamous epithelium with a keratotic surface. The basal cells are flat, unlike those in the primordial cyst. The keratotic layer is usually parakeratinized and tends to fill the cyst cavity (*Figs.* 20*a*, *b*). Midpalatine raphe cysts have a similar histological appearance (*Figs.* 21*a*, *b*).

Treatment

There is no indication for any treatment of gingival cysts in infants.

CHAPTER 4

GINGIVAL CYST OF ADULTS AND THE
LATERAL PERIODONTAL CYST

THERE is a great deal of confusion about the relationship between the gingival cyst of adults and the lateral periodontal cyst, much of which appears to have arisen because both types of cyst have a predilection for occurrence in the canine and premolar area of the mandible. The pathogenesis of these cysts, particularly with regard to the cells of origin, is also far from clear. This confusion is further complicated by the fact that many cysts in the lateral periodontal position are really primordial cysts (Soskolne and Shear, 1967), while others are of inflammatory origin arising adjacent to an accessory root canal in the presence of a necrotic pulp, or by infection through the gingival crevice. Bhaskar (1965) grouped the gingival and lateral periodontal cysts together as gingival cysts and considered that they both arise from extraosseous odontogenic epithelium although 13 of his 29 cases showed circumscribed radiolucencies indicative of lateral periodontal cysts. He believed that the radiolucencies were the result of cup-shaped depressions on the periosteal surfaces of the cortical plates produced by enlargement of the gingival cysts.

On the other hand, other workers (Shafer et al., 1974) and Shear and Pindborg (1975) were of the opinion that the two are not related and should be differentiated from one another. The gingival cysts may certainly occur without bone involvement and may produce a gingival swelling although usually they go unnoticed and most of them have been detected in the course of histological examination of large numbers of gingival biopsies (Moskow, 1966). Ritchey and Orban (1953) discovered 6 such cysts in 350 gingival biopsies. It is improbable, though not impossible, that a cyst originating in the gingival soft tissues could enlarge sufficiently to produce a radiologically obvious bone erosion without producing any gingival swelling. Yet many lateral periodontal cysts are discovered on routine radiological examination in the absence of any clinical symptoms or signs (Moskow et al., 1970; Gold and Sliwkowski, 1973). These are likely to have arisen within the periodontal ligament and eroded outwards. In the case of lesions which have produced both gingival swelling and a radiolucency, however, it becomes impossible to determine the origin without surgical exploration. If such a procedure reveals that there is surface

31

erosion of cortical bone but no communication with the perio-dontium, then the diagnosis is gingival cyst. If there is communica-tion with the periodontium then the lesion is more likely to be a lateral periodontal cyst which has eroded outwards.

GINGIVAL CYST OF ADULTS
Clinical Features
The patient may give a history of a slowly enlarging swelling which is usually painless. The cysts are well-circumscribed, up to 1 cm diameter and may occur in the free, the attached gingiva, or the gingival papilla. The surface is smooth and may be bluish (*Fig. 22*).

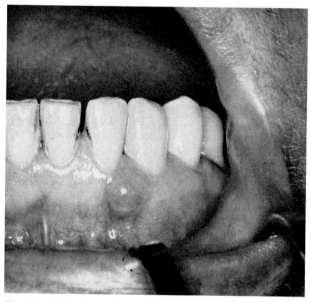

Fig. 22. Gingival cyst in an adult. (*Courtesy of Professor J. J. Pindborg.*)

The lesions are soft and fluctuant and the adjacent teeth are usually vital. Meaningful clinical data are not available as most published studies have combined gingival and lateral periodontal cysts. Moskow et al. (1970), for example, have surveyed the clinical data in 62 reported cases of gingival and lateral periodontal cysts and added 25 of their own. The mandible was involved in 68 of the 87 cases (78 per cent) and 49 of these were found between the canine and first premolar teeth. They occurred over a wide age distribution from the second to the eighth decades with a peak incidence in the fifth and sixth decades. They were slightly more frequent in males than in females (1·4 : 1). Of the 46 cases diagnosed as gingival cysts, 19 showed radiolucencies. The clinical data of Gold and Sliwkowski (1973), derived in the same way from a mixture of 26 gingival and lateral periodontal cysts and also 6 primordial cysts, were similar except that they showed a female predilection (2·6 : 1).

Pathogenesis

A number of suggestions have been made about the pathogenesis of the gingival cyst in adults. It has been proposed (Ritchey and Orban, 1953) that they may arise from odontogenic epithelial cell rests; or by traumatic implantation of surface epithelium; or by cystic degeneration of deep projections of surface epithelium. It has also been postulated that, very rarely, they may be derived from glandular elements (Traeger, 1961).

The most common origin is from odontogenic epithelial cell rests derived from the dental lamina although Shafer et al. (1974) felt that cysts arising from traumatic implantation of surface epithelium may occur. Reference has already been made to the frequency with which remnants of the dental lamina, many of them forming microcysts, are found in the gingivae of infants. In a study of 266 specimens of adult human gingiva, Stout et al. (1968) demonstrated epithelial rests in 90 and a true cyst in 1. They found no evidence of traumatic implantation or heterotopic glandular tissue. Many of the epithelial remnants which they observed resembled the cell rests of Malassez. Hodson (1962) found epithelial residues in the anterior incisor areas in 58 per cent of 26 autopsies and in 14 per cent of 58 edentulous third molar regions. In a number of cases cell rests were found in the connective tissue of the gum without any specific relation to the surface epithelium. Unfortunately, for purposes of the present discussion, Hodson did not examine mandibular premolar regions. There is no clear explanation as to what the stimulus for the proliferation of these rests and their subsequent cystic breakdown might be, but it is certainly not an inflammatory stimulus which produces well-recognized effects on odontogenic epithelium in radicular cysts, as are described in Chapter 11.

Histology

Gingival cysts in the adult have a variable histological pattern. They are usually small. Some have an extremely thin epithelium with one or two layers of flat cells containing darkly-staining nuclei. In others the epithelial lining may be of a rather thicker stratified squamous nature (*Figs. 23a, b*). A parakeratotic layer may be found on the surface of the epithelium and keratotic cells may be found in the cyst lumen. Bhaskar (1965) has referred to the presence in these

33

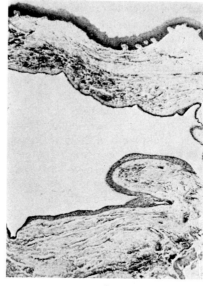

a

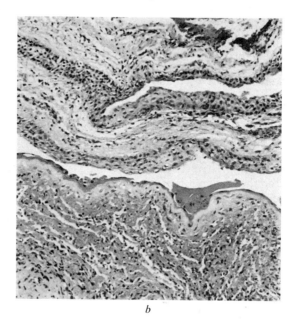

b

Fig. 23*a*, Gingival cyst in an adult. The cyst lies deep to gingival epithelium. It is lined partly by a thin epithelial lining 1–2 cell layers wide and partly by a thicker stratified squamous epithelium. HE; ×24. *b*, Gingival cyst in an adult. Another case showing a folded epithelial lining of varying thickness. Some discontinuities are also present. HE; ×110.

cysts of epithelial thickenings consisting of fusiform or 'water clear' cells forming a pavement-like arrangement. These epithelial thickenings or plaques certainly occur in lateral periodontal cysts (Shear and Pindborg, 1975). In view of the difficulty often encountered in differentiating clinically between adult gingival and lateral periodontal cysts, it is not certain whether they do in fact also occur in the former. They may well do so, but histological descriptions of series in which the two categories of cyst are clearly distinguished clinically, are necessary before this question can be answered definitely. Other fragments of odontogenic epithelium may be present adjacent to the cysts and irregular calcific fragments may also be found. The cysts are surrounded by the gingival connective tissue and there may be a variable degree of chronic inflammatory infiltrate.

Treatment

The gingival cyst can be removed by local surgical excision and there is no tendency for recurrence.

LATERAL PERIODONTAL CYST

Clinical Features

As published studies on the lateral periodontal cyst have usually included material on the gingival cyst of adults, there are inadequate data on age and sex distribution. It seems however that the lateral periodontal cysts occur most frequently in the canine-premolar area of the mandible and rarely occur before the age of 20 years. They are usually symptomless and are discovered fortuitously during routine radiological examination of the teeth. Occasionally a gingival swelling may occur and it is this type of case which must be differentiated from a gingival cyst. The associated teeth are usually vital unless they happen to have been otherwise involved.

Radiological Features

Radiographs of the lateral periodontal cyst show a well-defined round or ovid radiolucent area with a sclerotic margin. The cyst lies somewhere between the apex and the cervical margin of the tooth (*Fig.* 24). They vary in size from as small as 1 mm to larger lesions which may involve the entire length of a root.

Pathogenesis

Standish and Shafer (1958) commented that the lateral periodontal cyst was of varied aetiology but that the term 'lateral periodontal cyst' should be used to indicate all cysts developing in the anatomic region of the lateral periodontium. In view of this varied aetiology however, they suggested that the term should be qualified to indicate whether the cyst's origin is pulp infection, infection through the gingival crevice or idiopathic stimulation of cell rests. In my opinion, however, the term 'lateral periodontal cyst' should be confined to cysts in the lateral periodontal position in which an inflammatory

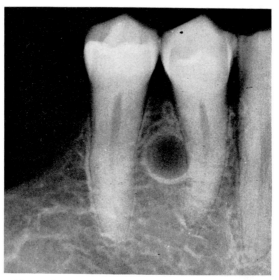

Fig. 24. Radiograph of lateral periodontal cyst between the mandibular premolar teeth. Primordial cysts also sometimes occur in this situation and in such cases are indistinguishable radiologically from lateral periodontal cysts.

*(Figs. 24, 26, 27 and 28 were previously published (1975) in Scand. J. Dent. Res. **83**, 103–110, and are reproduced here by courtesy of the Editor.)*

aetiology and a diagnosis of collateral primordial cyst have been excluded on clinical and histological grounds (Shear and Pindborg, 1975).

Although there can be little doubt that lateral periodontal cysts are of odontogenic origin, there is, as with many other odontogenic lesions, considerable doubt as to precisely which odontogenic epithelium they arise from. Proof of origin from any particular source is lacking and any hypotheses must therefore be based on presumptive evidence. Histological studies show that they are usually devoid of inflammatory cell infiltration except at a distance from the lining and it is reasonable therefore to regard them as being of developmental origin.

Assuming then that the lateral periodontal cyst is a distinct entity of developmental odontogenic origin, how does it arise? The available evidence suggests two possibilities.

As may also be seen from a description of the histological features, it is lined for the most part by a narrow non-keratinized epithelium which resembles reduced enamel epithelium. As such, the proposal that it arises initially as a dentigerous cyst developing by expansion

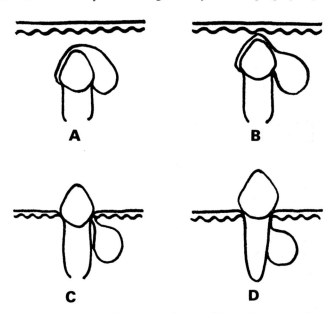

A　　　　　**B**

C　　　　　**D**

Fig. 25. Diagram illustrating the possible pathogenesis of a lateral periodontal cyst. At A there is expansion of the follicle on the lateral surface of the crown of an unerupted tooth. At this stage a radiograph would show a lateral dentigerous cyst. At B–D the tooth erupts leaving the expanded follicle behind.

of the follicle along the lateral surface of the crown (Shafer et al., 1974), is an attractive one. *Fig.* 34 (p. 48) is a radiograph of such a phenomenon, which is usually referred to as a lateral dentigerous cyst. If tooth eruption is normal, the expanded follicle may finally lie on the lateral aspect of the root, as illustrated diagrammatically in *Fig.* 25. This hypothesis is supported by the fact that lateral periodontal cysts tend to occur in areas where dentigerous cysts are commonly located. In this respect it is of interest that epithelial plaques similar to those seen in the lateral periodontal cyst are sometimes found in dentigerous cysts.

The second possibility is origin from the cell rests of Malassez. There is no clue however as to the stimulus which produces this

37

type of proliferation in the Malassez rests nor what might be responsible for their cystic breakdown. Where islands of odontogenic epithelium are seen in the wall of a lateral periodontal cyst as they sometimes are, it is quite possible that these are remnants of the dental lamina and that the lateral periodontal cyst, having broken through the alveolar plate, now lies close to them.

Histology

Most commonly the lateral periodontal cyst is lined by a thin, non-keratinizing layer of squamous or cuboidal epithelium usually ranging from one to five cell layers thick which resembles the reduced enamel epithelium (*Fig. 26*). The epithelial cells are sometimes

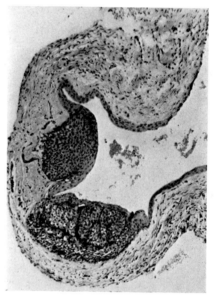

Fig. 26. Lateral periodontal cyst which in part has a thin non-keratinized stratified squamous epithelial lining resembling reduced enamel epithelium. Two epithelial plaques are seen. The lower of these is convoluted as in stage F in *Fig. 28*. HE; × 50.

separated by intercellular fluid. Their nuclei are small and pyknotic. Sometimes the epithelial lining may be of a more distinctly stratified squamous nature. When, however, it has the characteristic features of a primordial cyst, then this should be the diagnosis rather than lateral periodontal cyst. Indeed, Gold and Sliwkowski (1973) have shown in their study that such collateral primordial cysts have, as one would expect, a definite tendency to recur following surgical removal.

An interesting feature which is seen in many lateral periodontal cysts is the presence of what appear to be localized plaques or thickenings of the epithelial lining (*Figs.* 26, 27, 28). Some of these are small whereas others are larger and extend into the surrounding cyst wall as well as producing mural bulges which protrude into the cyst cavity. Some cysts contain a number of the plaques. The cells of the plaque are sometimes fusiform with their long axes parallel to the basement membrane; frequently they are large and clear, showing the features of intracellular oedema, and contain small pyknotic nuclei.

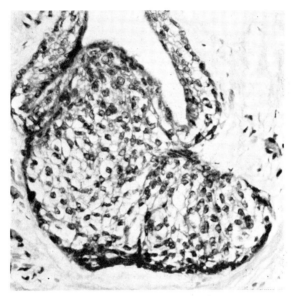

Fig. 27. Epithelial plaque in a lateral periodontal cyst. This is represented diagrammatically by stage E in *Fig.* 28. HE; ×225.

Examination of histological material at the light microscope level, and particularly study of serial sections, indicates the possible mode of formation of these plaques (Shear and Pindborg, 1975). The usual sequence (*Fig.* 28) is that there appears to be proliferation of the flat basal cells which produces a slight localized thickening of the epithelium. At this stage the thickened epithelium consists predominantly of darkly staining fusiform basal cells. This early plaque may extend into the fibrous wall of the cyst or bulge into the lumen. The plaque increases in size both by further basal cell proliferation and by swelling of these epithelial cells. At this stage there is a more pronounced bulging into the lumen and also into

39

the wall. The bulbous nature of the thickening into the wall some-times leads to undermining of the adjacent cyst lining. Complex convolutions of the epithelium may be seen in the larger plaques. Occasionally the cells of the plaque may differentiate and take on a distinctly spinous appearance.

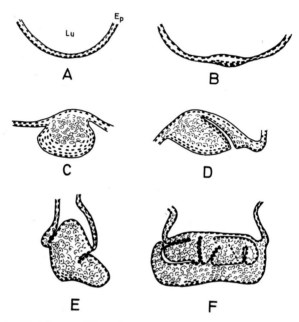

Fig. 28. Diagram illustrating the possible mode of formation of epithelial plaques by localized proliferation of cells. A, Cyst lined by thin epithelium resembling reduced enamel epithelium. B, Early epithelial thickening by basal cell proliferation. C, Basal cells continue to proliferate. Superficial cells swell by accumulation of intracellular fluid. D and E, Basal cell proliferation ceases or slows down. Superficial cells waterlogged and swollen. Plaque protrudes into cyst cavity and cyst wall. Can undermine and raise adjacent cyst lining. F, Epithelial plaque can form convolutions. Lu, Cyst lumen. Ep, Epithelial lining.

What produces these localized epithelial proliferations is not known. It does however seem to be a spontaneous process which tends to occur in reduced enamel epithelium and probably also in other lesions of odontogenic epithelium. It is possible that the thickenings represent another of the many examples of odontogenic epithelium recapitulating ontogeny under pathological conditions. In this instance, the process seems to be similar to that which takes place during the early stages of tooth development, when there is thickening of stomodeal ectoderm to form the dental lamina.

The cysts may be unilocular or there may be two or more locules. Thin-walled unilocular examples may collapse and fold and might, in some planes of section, appear bi- or multilocular. Sometimes a lesion may actually be multilocular and as such may be similar to, if not identical with, the so-called botryoid odontogenic cyst described below.

Islands of odontogenic epithelium are sometimes found in the cyst walls and some of them may also form microcysts.

The epithelial linings may separate to differing degrees from the fibrous cyst wall and there are occasional areas of juxta-epithelial hyalinized collagen. The fibrous cyst wall shows a variable chronic inflammatory cell infiltrate and is usually remarkably free of inflammation.

Grand and Marwah (1964) have reported a lateral periodontal cyst in a Negro, in the epithelial lining of which were melanin-containing cells.

Treatment

The lateral periodontal cyst is treated by surgical enucleation, after which it does not recur. Attempts should be made to avoid sacrificing the associated tooth, but this may not always be possible.

BOTRYOID ODONTOGENIC CYST

Weathers and Waldron (1973) have reported two examples of a multilocular cystic lesion of the jaws for which they proposed the term 'botryoid odontogenic cyst' because the gross specimen resembles a cluster of grapes. This may be a variant of the lateral periodontal cyst as there are radiological and histological similarities. Microscopically the lesion is multilocular with very thin fibrous connective tissue septa. The cyst cavities are lined by a compressed epithelium only 1–2 cells wide and there are foci of plaque-like thickenings consisting of swollen clear epithelial cells similar to those found in the lateral periodontal cyst. Weathers and Waldron suggested that these thickenings may possibly be the source of additional cyst locules.

CHAPTER 5

DENTIGEROUS (FOLLICULAR) CYST

A DENTIGEROUS cyst is one which encloses the crown of an unerupted tooth and is attached to the neck (*Fig. 29*). It is important that this definition be applied strictly and that the diagnosis of dentigerous cyst is not made on radiographic evidence, otherwise primordial cysts of the envelopmental variety (Main, 1970a) and unilocular

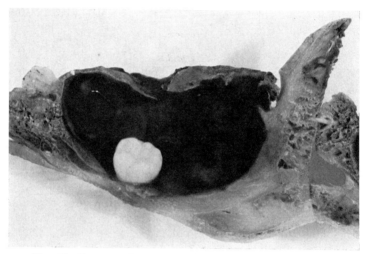

Fig. 29. Gross specimen of a dentigerous cyst involving the mandibular third molar tooth.

ameloblastomas involving adjacent unerupted teeth are liable to be misdiagnosed as dentigerous cysts.

Clinical Features

Frequency
In the 15-year period 1958–73, 103 of 750 jaw cysts accessioned in our department have been dentigerous cysts (13·7 per cent). This means that we are seeing about 7 cases a year and, as our material is drawn from a number of sources, individual surgeons and departments are apparently dealing with far fewer than this number each year.

Age

The age distribution of 91 cases in our series is shown in *Fig.* 30. Dentigerous cysts occur with a greater frequency than any other cyst, in the first decade. The incidence in the first decade is nevertheless lower than in the subsequent three decades. This is because the lower wisdom teeth and the maxillary permanent canines which are the teeth most frequently involved in dentigerous cysts are at an

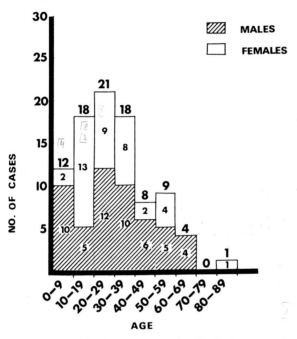

Fig. 30. Age distribution of 91 patients with dentigerous cysts.

early stage of development (*Fig.* 31). Of 12 cases in the first decade, the mandibular first premolar was involved in 4, the mandibular second premolar and first permanent molar twice each, and the maxillary permanent central, lateral, canine and first premolar were involved once. In the second decade, there is a higher incidence than in the first, most of the cysts involving the lower wisdom and the upper permanent canine. The third and fourth decades show the peak involvement of the lower wisdom teeth and it is during the third decade that the upper wisdom tooth becomes involved for the first time. During the subsequent decades there is a gradual decline in incidence with the mandibular wisdoms and maxillary permanent canines most frequently involved.

43

It is interesting to observe that the age distribution in our South African sample is similar to that of Mourshed's (1964c) United States group, whereas the British material of Killey and Kay (1972) and Browne (1972) shows a peak incidence at a later age. A difference in age distribution of radicular cysts between British and South African samples has also been observed and is commented on under that heading.

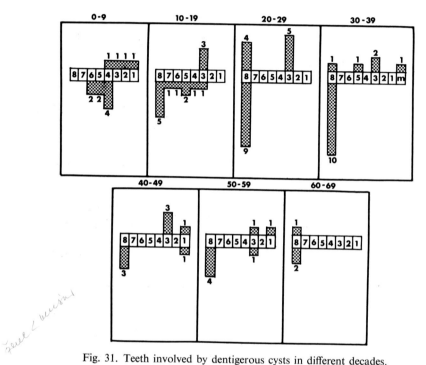

Fig. 31. Teeth involved by dentigerous cysts in different decades.

Sex (Table 5)
The incidence of dentigerous cysts is greater in males than females (P<5 per cent). Of 97 patients in our sample for whom this information is available, 59 (61 per cent) were males and 38 (29 per cent) females, a male : female ratio of 1·6 : 1. These figures are almost identical to those of Mourshed's United States sample although the series of both Browne and Killey and Kay show an even greater male preponderance.

Although there might be a tendency to assume that the less frequent occurrence in females results from their having a lower incidence of unerupted teeth, this assumption is not borne out by data such as that collected by Mourshed (1964a). In a survey of an unselected sample of full-mouth radiographs, he found that there was no sex difference in the incidence of unerupted teeth. This suggests that there is another factor, as yet not identified, which may influence the development of these cysts other than the mere physical fact of their origin in unerupted teeth.

Table 5.
SEX DISTRIBUTION OF BLACK AND WHITE PATIENTS WITH DENTIGEROUS CYSTS

	Male	Female	Total	M : F ratio
Black	11	4	15	2·8 : 1
White	48	34	82	1·4 : 1
Total	59 (61%)	38 (39%)	97	1·6 : 1
W : B ratio	4·4 : 1	8·5 : 1	5·5 : 1	

Race (Table 5)

In our material there is a very much higher incidence of dentigerous cysts in Whites than in Blacks. Of 97 patients, 82 were Whites and 15 were Blacks, a ratio of 5·5 : 1. As the population on the Witwatersrand from which the sample is collected is predominantly Black (1·6 : 1) it seems that Blacks have a lesser tendency than Whites to develop dentigerous cysts. In Mourshed's series, there was also a very considerable preponderance of White patients compared with Negroes, but Mourshed discounted this on the grounds that the biopsy service at his School deals predominantly with material from White patients.

If, however, the difference in racial incidence is a real one, then the reason for this must be sought either in parallel differences in the incidence of impacted teeth or in the unidentified factor which may be responsible for the greater preponderance in males than females. No data are available for the incidence of impacted teeth in South African Blacks compared with Whites, but Jacobson (1967) has studied the crania of 460 South African Blacks. He found that 75 per cent of males and females had sufficient space to accommodate all teeth in the maxilla and about 64 per cent of both male and female could accommodate all teeth in the mandible. A study of 139 Caucasoid children aged 13 years (Lundström, 1960) showed that teeth were crowded in 40 per cent. These differences are insufficient to explain the disparity in distribution of dentigerous cysts in the two racial groups.

Site

The anatomical distribution of 78 dentigerous cysts, in relation to tooth involved, is shown in *Fig.* 32 and this has already been discussed with regard to the age distribution. A very substantial majority involve the mandibular third molar. We find that the maxillary permanent canine is next in order of frequency of involvement, followed by the maxillary third molar and the mandibular premolars.

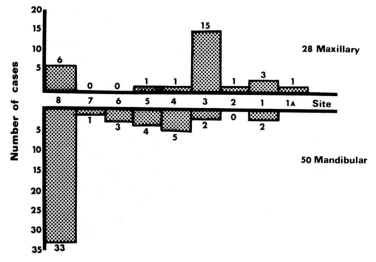

Fig. 32. Anatomical distribution of 78 dentigerous cysts.

Clinical Presentation

Like primordial cysts, dentigerous cysts may grow to a large size before they are diagnosed. Most of them are discovered on radiographs when these are taken because a tooth has failed to erupt, or a tooth is missing, or because teeth are tilted or are otherwise out of alignment. Many patients first become aware of the cysts because of slowly enlarging swellings, and this is the common form of presentation with edentulous patients in whose jaws unerupted teeth have inadvertently been retained. Dentigerous cysts may occasionally be painful particularly if infected. Although patients may give a history of slowly-enlarging swelling, Seward (1964) has shown radiologically that lesions 4–5 cm in diameter may develop in 3–4 years.

Radiological Features

Radiographs show unilocular radiolucent areas associated with the crowns of unerupted teeth. The cysts have well-defined sclerotic

46

margins unless they become infected, when the margins are poorly defined. Occasionally trabeculations may be seen and this may give an erroneous impression of multilocularity. The unerupted teeth may be impacted as a result of inadequate space in the dental arch or as a result of malpositioning such as by a horizontally impacted mandibular third molar or an inverted tooth. A supernumerary tooth may develop a dentigerous cyst (Mourshed, 1964b).

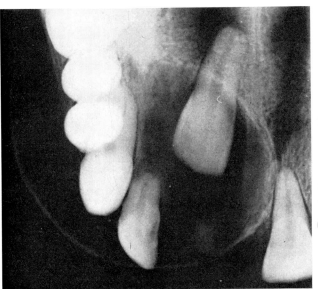

Fig. 33. Radiograph of a central type dentigerous cyst involving a maxillary canine tooth. (*Courtesy of Dr M. Copelyn.*)

The most common relationship of the cyst to the unerupted crown is central or coronal (*Fig.* 33). Here the crown is enveloped symmetrically. In these instances, pressure is applied to the crown of the tooth and may push it away from its direction of eruption. In this way, mandibular third molars may be found at the lower border of the mandible or in the ascending ramus and a maxillary canine may be forced into the maxillary sinus as far as the floor of the orbit, or it may be found below the floor of the nose. The lateral type of dentigerous cyst (*Fig.* 34) is a radiographic appearance which results from dilatation of the follicle on one aspect of the crown. This type is commonly seen when an impacted mandibular third molar is partially erupted so that its superior aspect is exposed. The lateral dentigerous cyst is seen on the inferior aspect of the tooth. The so-called circumferential dentigerous cyst in which the

47

entire tooth appears to be enveloped by cyst (*Fig.* 35) is probably an envelopmental type of primordial cyst in some cases, although it is

–cerae was folu –
impulcacis ube;

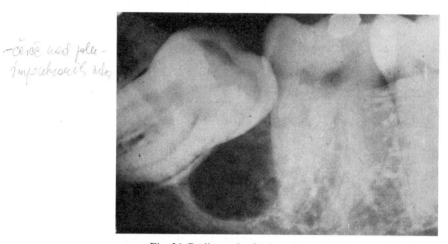

Fig. 34. Radiograph of a lateral type dentigerous cyst.

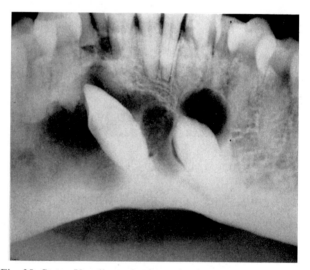

Fig. 35. Status X radiograph of two dentigerous cysts. The cyst on the right is a lateral type; that on the left is a circumferential type.

possible that a follicle may expand in such a way that it would appear radiographically as if the entire tooth was 'floating' in the cyst (*Fig.* 36).

48

Some unerupted teeth have a slightly dilated follicle in the pre-eruptive phase. This does not signify a cyst, nor even necessarily a potential cyst unless the pericoronal width is at least 3–4 mm.

Dentigerous cysts appear to have a greater tendency than other simple jaw cysts to produce some resorption of the roots of adjacent teeth (Struthers and Shear, 1976).

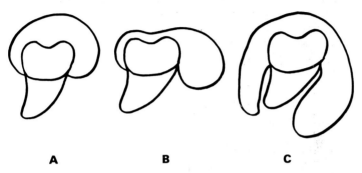

A　　　　**B**　　　　**C**

Fig. 36. Diagram illustrating the manner in which the dental follicle may expand to produce the radiographic appearances of A, central; B, lateral; and C, circumferential type dentigerous cysts.

Pathogenesis

There can be little doubt that dentigerous cysts develop around the crowns of unerupted teeth, whatever causes the latter to fail to erupt. In an analysis of the distribution of 761 unerupted teeth in 304 patients, Mourshed (1964a) showed that the vast majority (706) were mandibular or maxillary third molars. Maxillary canines were next, a long way behind (15), followed by mandibular second premolars (11), maxillary second molars (8), mandibular second molars (7), mandibular canines (6) and maxillary second molars (4). The mandibular and maxillary first premolars, a maxillary central incisor and a supernumerary tooth were each involved once. There is clearly some correlation between these figures and the incidence of dentigerous cysts, although it would appear from the respective proportions that an unerupted maxillary canine seems to have a greater risk of developing a dentigerous cyst than the mandibular third molar, which in turn has a greater risk than the maxillary third molar. Mourshed (1964a) has calculated that the incidence of dentigerous cysts is 1·44 in every 100 unerupted teeth. Toller's estimate (1967) was that possibly 1 in 150 unerupted teeth might develop a dentigerous cyst, and the risk seems to be greater in individuals over 30 years than in those who are younger. The anatomical environment of an unerupted tooth is probably of some significance in determining the development of a cyst. As I have

49

mentioned before, however, the differences in sex and race incidence do suggest that there is some other factor, as yet unidentified, which may play some role in determining whether a cyst will develop.

It has been suggested that dentigerous cysts may be of either extrafollicular or intrafollicular origin and that those of intra-follicular origin may develop by accumulation of fluid either between the reduced enamel epithelium and the enamel, or within the enamel organ itself. I am inclined to reject the extrafollicular theory as cysts which have been reported as arising in this manner appear to be envelopmental primordial. The case reported by Gillette and Weinmann (1958) and which is frequently quoted in support of extrafollicular origin, is clearly an envelopmental primordial cyst (*Fig.* 8, p. 15). Occasional dentigerous cyst linings show projections which resemble Tomes' processes of the ameloblasts protruding into the lumen from the superficial layer of epithelial cells. This suggests that in these instances the superficial cells were derived from the ameloblasts and provides evidence that at least in some cases, dentigerous cysts arise by accumulation of fluid between the reduced enamel epithelium and the enamel, and not in the stellate reticulum.

Another theory of origin which has been proposed is that the crown of a permanent tooth may erupt into a radicular cyst of its deciduous predecessor. Although this is a theoretical possibility, it must be exceptionally rare if only because radicular cysts involving the deciduous dentition are so uncommon. In such a case the erupting tooth would indent rather than penetrate the wall of the radicular cyst and this should be apparent histologically, if not macroscopically.

Presuming then that the dentigerous cyst develops around an unerupted tooth by accumulation of fluid between the reduced enamel epithelium and the enamel, how does this happen? Main (1970b) suggested that the pressure exerted by a potentially-erupting tooth on an impacted follicle obstructs the venous outflow and thereby induces rapid transudation of serum across the capillary walls. The increased hydrostatic pressure of this pooling fluid separates the follicle from the crown, with or without reduced enamel epithelium. With time, capillary permeability is altered so as to permit the passage of greater quantities of protein above the low concentration of the pure transudate. Main made the point that the pooling fluid separates the follicle from the crown, with or without reduced enamel epithelium, on the basis of the work of Stanley et al. (1965) who studied 70 non-cystic follicles from the third molars of patients ranging in age from 13 to 69 years. They concluded that follicles separated from enamel in patients below 22 years of age tend to leave the still-cuboidal reduced enamel

50

epithelium attached to tooth, while above this age the progressively more squamous epithelium becomes increasingly more readily detached. The frequent occurrence of 'epithelial discontinuities' described by Toller (1966a) in about one-third of uninfected dentigerous cysts suggests that in some of these cysts the reduced enamel epithelium may separate in parts and adhere to the enamel in other parts.

Many dentigerous cysts show evidence of acute and chronic inflammation in their walls, and in these instances exudation must play some part in the expansion of the cyst. Moreover, the passage of desquamated epithelial cells and inflammatory cells into the cyst cavity must contribute to the increase in intracystic osmotic tension and thereby probably to further expansion of the cyst. Toller (1970b) has shown that the mean cyst fluid osmolality of 7 dentigerous cysts was 10 milliosmoles higher than the mean serum osmolality but that this increase was not statistically significant. He believed (Toller, 1967) that the likely origin of dentigerous cysts is a breakdown of proliferating cells of the follicle following impeded eruption. Although he conceded that the factors favouring fluid accumulation which were postulated by Main may possibly play a role, he believed that raised osmolality of the cyst fluid plays an important role in the cyst expansion.

A possibly useful experimental model for the study of the pathogenesis of dentigerous cysts has been developed by Riviere and Sabet (1973). They transplanted unerupted molar tooth germs from 7-day-old mice to the mammary fat pads of adult mice of the same inbred line. Cysts with a dentigerous relationship to the crown of the tooth developed in every instance that the graft retained its viability and they developed at about the same rate in all animals over a 3-week period.

Pathology

Sometimes the cyst is removed intact but more often the thin wall is torn during the surgical procedure. Pathologists should do a careful dissection of the gross specimen to determine that the cyst surrounding the crown of the tooth is indeed a dilated follicle and that it attaches at the amelocemental junction. Some primordial cysts may appear, in the gross specimen, to be a dentigerous cyst, and on opening into such a cyst an intact follicle will be revealed. In an inflamed dentigerous cyst the wall may be thickened.

Histological examination usually shows a thin fibrous cyst wall which, being derived from dental follicle, consists of young fibroblasts widely separated by stroma and ground substance rich in acid mucopolysaccharide. The epithelial lining, which is in fact reduced enamel epithelium, consists of 2–3 cell layers of flat or cuboidal cells

51

(*Fig.* 37). Characteristically, the epithelial lining is not keratinized and most of those which have been described as keratinized have usually been primordial. Very rarely, a dentigerous cyst lining may apparently form keratin by metaplasia (*Fig.* 38). Discontinuities in the epithelial lining may be seen in the presence of an intense inflammatory infiltrate in the adjacent capsule, or, as suggested by Toller (1966a) through partial adherence to enamel. Sometimes, the superficial layer of the epithelial lining is low columnar and retains the morphology of the ameloblast layer which of course, it originally was.

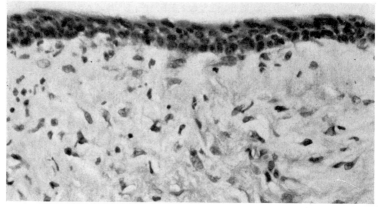

Fig. 37. Wall of a dentigerous cyst lined by a thin epithelium derived from the reduced enamel epithelium. HE; ×250.

In some cysts part of the epithelial lining may contain mucus-producing cells. Browne (1972) found them in 36 per cent of mandibular and in 53 per cent of maxillary dentigerous cysts in his series, and made the interesting observation that the incidence of such mucus cells increased in proportion to the age of the patients. Ciliated cells occur very rarely. The presence of these mucus and ciliated cells are thought to result from metaplasia. Another rare example of metaplasia in dentigerous cysts is provided by the occasional presence of sebaceous glands in their walls (Gorlin, 1957; Spouge, 1966). Hyaline bodies (Rushton, 1955) are seen occasionally.

Localized proliferation of epithelial lining may occur in response to inflammation. Occasional bud-like thickenings of the epithelium may be seen in the absence of inflammation and sometimes there may be budding of the basal cells into the fibrous capsule. Nests, islands and strands of odontogenic epithelium are often seen in the capsule.

The Dentigerous Cyst as a Potential Ameloblastoma
A number of workers have claimed that many ameloblastomas arise in dentigerous cysts but I have seen no evidence to support such a contention. Indeed, the fact that dentigerous cysts are so rare in South African Blacks, compared with Whites, whereas ameloblastomas are five times more common in Blacks (Meerkotter, 1969), provides contrary evidence. While ameloblastomas, being of odontogenic epithelial origin, may of course theoretically arise from

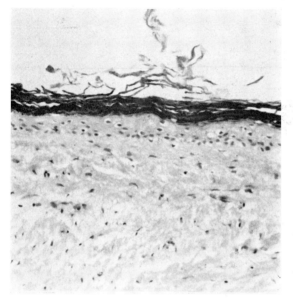

Fig. 38. Keratinizing epithelium lining a dentigerous cyst. HE; ×185.

dentigerous cyst lining as well as any other odontogenic epithelium, the belief that it commonly arises in this situation and that the dentigerous cyst should therefore be regarded as pre-ameloblastomatous, should be viewed with caution. Much of the confusion has, I believe, arisen for three reasons. Firstly, an ameloblastoma, like a primordial cyst, may involve an unerupted tooth, particularly a third molar at the angle of the mandible, and this may be incorrectly interpreted as a dentigerous cyst on radiographs (*Fig. 39*). When subsequently the lesion is removed and diagnosed histologically as an ameloblastoma, the erroneous conclusion may be reached that the ameloblastoma developed from the dentigerous cyst.

The second possible reason for believing that many ameloblastomas develop from dentigerous cysts is that biopsies of ameloblastomas are often taken of an expanded locule lined apparently by a thin layer of epithelium. If the surgeon's provisional diagnosis is dentigerous cyst because of the radiological picture, the pathologist may well regard such histological features as consistent with the diagnosis. When the tumour is removed entirely and a diagnosis of ameloblastoma is made, once again this may be misinterpreted as having developed from a dentigerous cyst. Thirdly, as Lucas (1954) has pointed out, apparently isolated islets or follicles of epithelium are sometimes found in the cyst wall some distance from the

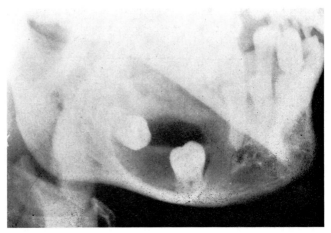

Fig. 39. Ameloblastoma with the radiological appearance of a dentigerous cyst.

epithelial lining. These have been interpreted as ameloblastoma although they bear only a superficial resemblance to the tumour.

I have seen an interesting case in Professor Pindborg's collection. The lesion was a dentigerous cyst with a mural nodule which consisted of tissue very similar to that of a plexiform ameloblastoma. The entire ameloblastoma-like mass protruded into the cyst cavity and there was no evidence of any tumour infiltration of the cyst wall (*Fig.* 40). The question arises therefore whether this mass can be regarded as an ameloblastoma if it does not behave like one. Whether it is or not, it must be emphasized that this phenomenon is a definite rarity.

Treatment

When a dentigerous cyst has developed around a mandibular third molar, the treatment is usually careful enucleation together with the involved tooth. In children, Killey and Kay (1972) strongly recommend marsupialization when the involved tooth and possibly adjacent teeth are prevented from assuming their normal position in the arch. Their experience is that if the operation is done during the eruptive phase of the involved teeth, these will probably erupt

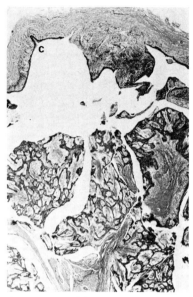

Fig. 40. Dentigerous cyst with mural nodule consisting of tissue very similar to that of a plexiform ameloblastoma. C=cyst lining. (*Section lent by Professor J. J. Pindborg.*) HE; ×20.

and come into a functional occlusion as the cyst cavity fills with new bone. If they do not erupt properly, they can be removed at a later stage.

55

CHAPTER 6

ERUPTION CYST

AN eruption cyst is in fact a dentigerous cyst occurring in the soft tissues. Whereas the dentigerous cyst develops around the crown of an unerupted tooth lying in the bone, the eruption cyst occurs when a tooth is impeded in its eruption within the soft tissues overlying the bone.

Clinical Features

Frequency

Eruption cysts are not common and only 7 have been seen in our Department in 15 years (0·9 per cent). It is possible that they occur more frequently clinically and that as some burst spontaneously these are not excised and are therefore not submitted for histological examination. Six of the 7 cysts were in White male children aged 1, 1, 6, 7, 7 and 9 years and involved, respectively, $\overline{|D}$, $\overline{D|}$, $\overline{6|}$, $\overline{4|}$, $\overline{1|1}$, and $|\overline{4}$. The seventh patient was a female aged 46 with delayed eruption of $\overline{1|}$. Seward (1973) reported on the features of 7 cases and also reviewed the literature. In her material the ages of the patients ranged from newborn infants to 21 years and there was a preponderance of females (2 : 1).

Clinical Presentation

The eruption cyst produces a smooth swelling over the erupting tooth which may be either the colour of normal gingiva, or blue (*Fig.* 41). It is usually painless unless infected. It is soft and fluctuant.

Sometimes more than one cyst may be present. There is often a brief history of about 3–4 weeks' duration during which they enlarge to approximately 1–1·5 cm. They are usually exposed to masticatory trauma. Transillumination is a useful diagnostic aid in distinguishing an eruption cyst from an eruption haematoma (Seward, 1973).

Radiological Features

The cyst may throw a soft-tissue shadow, but there is usually no bone involvement except that the dilated and open crypt may be seen on the radiograph.

Pathogenesis

The pathogenesis of the eruption cyst is probably very similar to that of the dentigerous cyst. The difference is that the tooth in the case of the eruption cyst is impeded in the soft tissues of the gingivae rather than in the bone. The factors which actually impede eruption in the soft tissues are not known, but the presence of particularly dense fibrous tissue could be responsible.

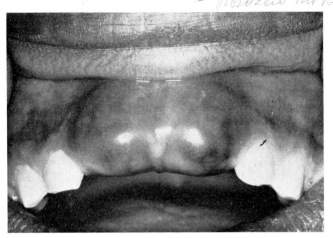

Fig. 41. Eruption cysts involving the permanent maxillary central incisors.

Pathology

As most eruption cysts are treated by marsupialization, the pathologist usually receives part of the cyst wall. The superficial aspect is covered by the keratinized stratified squamous epithelium of the overlying gingiva. This is separated from the cyst by a strip of dense connective tissue of varying thickness which usually shows a mild chronic inflammatory cell infiltrate. As the cysts are so frequently exposed to masticatory trauma the inflammatory infiltrate invariably increases in intensity towards the cyst lining, adjacent to which it is most intense. Sometimes it is possible to distinguish a line of demarcation between gingival and follicular connective tissues. The gingival connective tissue is relatively acellular and densely collagenous, and so has an eosinophilic hue. The follicular connective tissue is more densely cellular, less collagenous and has a more basophilic hue, presumably because of a higher content of acid mucopolysaccharide in the ground substance. Odontogenic epithelial cell rests may be present in the connective tissue.

In non-inflamed areas, the epithelial lining of the cyst is characteristically of reduced enamel epithelial origin, consisting in the main of 2–3 cell layers of squamous epithelium with a few foci where it may be a little thicker. Invariably however the epithelial lining is intensely inflamed. Acute inflammatory cells are found in the epithelium which proliferates in response to the inflammatory

57

stimulus, and may form characteristic arcades. Such epithelium is grossly spongiotic. The adjacent corium is hyperaemic and the seat of a chronic inflammatory cell infiltrate (*Fig.* 42).

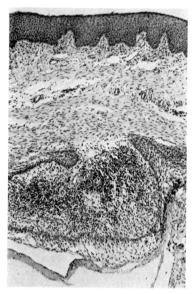

Fig. 42. Eruption cyst. The surface epithelium is at the top and the cyst epithelium at the bottom of the photomicrograph. HE; ×50.

Treatment

Eruption cysts are treated by marsupialization. The dome of the cyst is excised exposing the crown of the tooth, which is allowed to erupt.

CHAPTER 7

CALCIFYING ODONTOGENIC CYST

THE calcifying odontogenic cyst has many features of an odontogenic tumour and has in fact been classified as such by the World
Health Organization International Reference Centre for the Histological Definition and Classification of Odontogenic Tumours, Jaw
Cysts and Allied Lesions (Pindborg and Kramer, 1971). As a cyst,

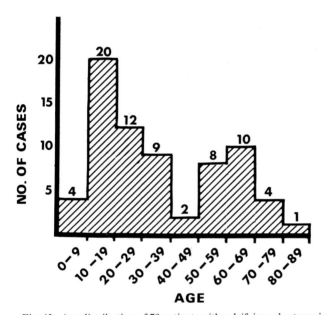

Fig. 43. Age distribution of 70 patients with calcifying odontogenic cysts.

it is probably best classified as of developmental odontogenic
epithelial origin. It was first described as a distinct entity by Gorlin
and associates (1962, 1964) who were impressed by its histological
resemblance to the cutaneous calcifying epithelioma of Malherbe.
Since then the lesion has been recognized in many pathology labora-
tories and a number of reports have appeared in the literature,
amongst which have been papers by Abrams and Howell (1968),
Ulmansky et al. (1969) and Fejerskov and Krogh (1972).

59

Clinical Features

Frequency

Despite the fact that the calcifying odontogenic cyst is now a well-recognized lesion, relatively few cases have been recorded in the literature. We see only one or two cases a year in our Department and regard the lesion as extremely rare. The age and sex distributions recorded below are derived from a literature review combined with 8 personally observed cases studied in our Department by Altini and Farman (1975).

Age

The age distribution of 70 cases is shown in *Fig.* 43. The lesion occurs over a wide range of ages. The youngest recorded patient was 6 years and the oldest 82 years, but there does seem to be a peak in the second decade.

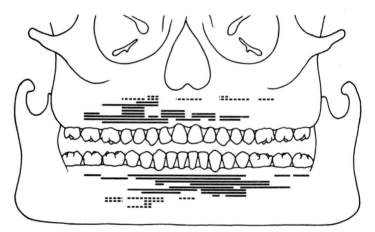

Fig. 44. Anatomical distribution of 50 cases of calcifying odontogenic cyst. (*Courtesy of Professor O. Fejerskov and the Editor,* Journal of Oral Pathology. *Previously published (1972) in* J. Oral Pathol. **1**, *273-287.*)

Sex

There is an almost equal distribution between male and female, so that of 69 cases, 33 were male and 36 female.

Race

No race predilection is apparent.

Site

The site distribution of 50 cases reported by Fejerskov and Krogh (1972) is illustrated in *Fig.* 44. The mandible (23 cases) and maxilla (27 cases) were involved with almost equal frequency. The majority

60

of cysts (36 cases) have occurred in the jaw bones and 15 have been found outside bone in the soft tissues related to the jaws. One case, recorded by Gorlin et al. (1964), occurred in the parotid salivary gland. It was surrounded by normal parotid tissue and was incompletely removed.

The most common site of occurrence has been the anterior part of the jaws. In the mandible, several cases have crossed the midline but this has been recorded in only two maxillary cases.

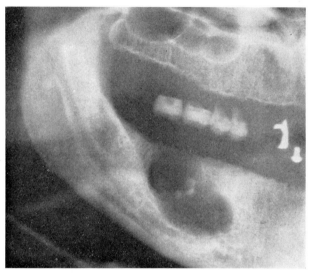

Fig. 45. Radiograph of a calcifying odontogenic cyst. The features of a radiolucent area with irregular radio-opacities are not specific. (*Courtesy of Dr. C. J. Nortjé*).

Clinical Presentation

Some patients have complained of swelling but only rarely has there been pain. Intraosseous lesions may produce a bony expansion and may be fairly extensive. Occasionally they may perforate the cortical plate and extend into the soft tissues. In a few cases displacement of the teeth has been described. A remarkably large number of cases have been completely symptomless and have been discovered fortuitously during routine radiological examination.

Radiological Features

The calcifying odontogenic cyst which occurs as an intraosseous lesion appears as an essentially radiolucent area. Some have a regular outline with well-demarcated margins. Others may be quite irregular and may have poorly defined margins. Some are unilocular

61

and others are multilocular lesions. Small irregular calcified bodies may be seen in the radiolucent area (*Fig.* 45) and in some cases the calcification may be substantial and occupy the greater part of the lesion. Dense opacities are likely to be present if the cyst is associated with a complex odontome, as it sometimes is. Some cases have been reported as being associated with an unerupted tooth. In a few cases resorption of the roots of adjacent teeth has occurred. Perforation of the cortical plate, when present, may be radiologically demonstrable.

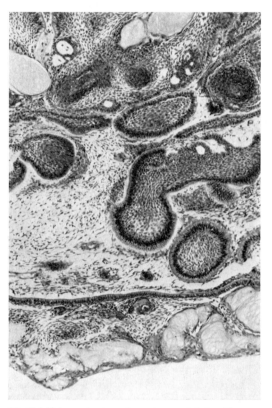

Fig. 46. Calcifying odontogenic cyst associated with an ameloblastic fibroma. HE; ×85.

It is clear from this description that the radiological picture is not diagnostic. Similar features of irregular calcifications in a radiolucent area may be exhibited by the ossifying fibroma, ameloblastic fibro-odontome, adenomatoid odontogenic tumour, calcifying epithelial odontogenic tumour and the odontoameloblastoma.

62

Pathogenesis and Pathology

The histological features of a classic calcifying odontogenic cyst are characteristic and present few diagnostic problems. Elucidation of the pathogenesis is however considerably complicated by the fact that the epithelial lining of a calcifying odontogenic cyst appears to have the ability to induce the formation of dental tissues in the adjacent connective tissue wall; and that other odontogenic tumours

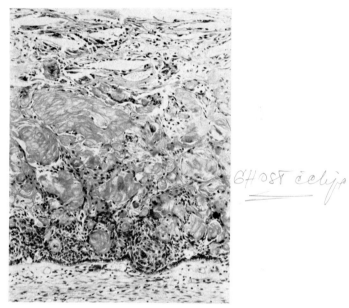

Fig. 47. Lining of a calcifying odontogenic cyst containing 'ghost cells'. The basal cells of the epithelium are columnar and have their nuclei orientated away from the basement membrane. HE; ×72.

such as the ameloblastoma, the odontoameloblastoma, the ameloblastic fibroma (*Fig.* 46) and the ameloblastic fibro-odontome may sometimes be associated with a calcifying odontogenic cyst (Praetorius, 1975). Praetorius points out that the ghost cells which are so characteristic a feature of the calcifying odontogenic cyst also occur in other odontogenic cysts, the craniopharyngioma and the calcifying epithelioma of Malherbe, as well as in the other odontogenic tumours already mentioned. It is an intriguing question whether those calcifying odontogenic cysts which have other features of odontogenic tumours develop these secondarily, or whether they are themselves secondary phenomena in pre-existing odontogenic tumours.

63

The lesion may consist of a single large cyst or a number of smaller cysts. Sometimes the impression of multiple cysts is given by tangential sections of a folded cyst wall.

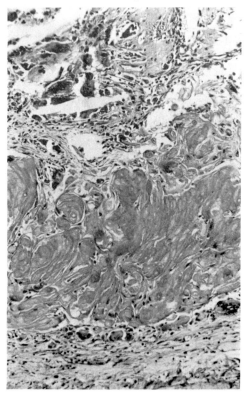

Fig. 48. 'Ghost cells' have broken through the epithelium and evoked a foreign body giant cell reaction. HE; ×80.

The epithelial lining has characteristic odontogenic features with a prominent basal layer consisting of columnar or cuboidal cells and hyperchromatic nuclei which are polarized away from the basement membrane (*Figs.* 46 and 47). The epithelium may be a regular 6–8 cells thick over part of its length and be continuous with parts which may be very thin and others which are considerably thickened.

The most remarkable feature of the calcifying odontogenic cyst is the presence of ghost cells which have been compared with those found in the calcifying epithelioma of Malherbe in the skin. These are found in groups, particularly in the thicker areas of the epithelial lining. The spinous cells in such situations may be widely separated by intercellular oedema and the epithelium around the ghost cells is often convoluted (*Figs.* 47 and 48).

The ghost cells consist of enlarged ballooned ovoid or elongated elliptoid epithelium. They are eosinophilic and although the cell outlines are usually well-defined, they may sometimes be blurred so that groups of them appear fused. A few ghost cells may contain nuclear remnants but these are in various stages of degeneration and in the majority all traces of chromatin have disappeared leaving only a faint outline of the original nucleus. The ghost cells represent

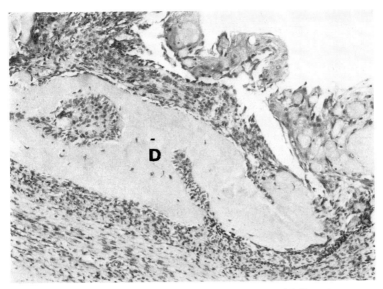

Fig. 49. Induction of dentinoid (D) adjacent to epithelium in a calcifying odontogenic cyst. HE; ×100.

an abnormal type of keratinization and have an affinity for calcification. They have the same histological reactions as keratin, giving a yellow fluorescence with Rhodamine B (Praetorius, 1975). Ultra-structurally, they do not show the same features as keratin in epidermis and oral epithelia (Fejerskov and Krogh, 1972) which are characterized by evenly distributed fine tonofilaments embedded in a matrix. The cytoplasm of some ghost cells in Fejerskov and Krogh's study contained fine tonofilaments separated by small empty spaces. Most of the cells showed very thick electron-dense fibre bundles of relatively uniform size which were sharply defined against the large empty spaces in the cytoplasm. Endoplasmic reticulum, mito-chondria, Golgi apparatus and ribosomes could not be identified. The cell membranes were intact with junctional complexes of various types.

65

The ghost cells may be in contact with the connective tissue wall of the cyst where they evoke a foreign-body reaction with the formation of multinucleate giant cells (*Fig.* 48). In the fibrous wall there are usually strands and islands of odontogenic epithelium, either in direct contact with the epithelium or separately in the connective tissue. These vary from a few strands to extensive proliferations.

An atubular dentinoid is usually found in the wall close to the epithelial lining and often in relation to the epithelial proliferations. It is frequently described as being found particularly in contact with masses of ghost cells (*Fig.* 49). I have seen a number of examples of calcifying odontogenic cyst with complex odontomes in their walls.

Melanin deposits are sometimes present in the epithelial linings.

Treatment

The calcifying odontogenic cyst is treated by surgical enucleation unless it is associated with another odontogenic tumour such as an ameloblastoma or an odontoameloblastoma, in which case the treatment will be more radical. Although classic uncomplicated cases may grow to a large size, reported recurrences are exceedingly rare.

CHAPTER 8

NASOPALATINE DUCT (INCISIVE CANAL) CYST

THE epithelial-lined cysts of non-odontogenic origin are thought to be derived from embryonic epithelial residues in the nasopalatine canal and, in the opinion of some workers, from epithelium included in lines of fusion of embryonic facial processes. The latter view is extremely controversial, as many embryologists and pathologists discount the possibility of such an origin.

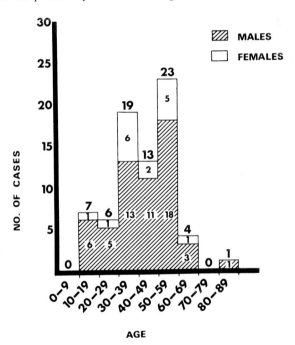

Fig. 50. Age distribution of 73 patients with nasopalatine duct cysts.

It is generally agreed that the nasopalatine duct cyst is an entity. It may occur within the nasopalatine canal or in the soft tissues of the palate, at the opening of the canal, where it is called the cyst of the palatine papilla. The term 'nasopalatine duct cyst' is preferred to the synonymous 'incisive canal cyst'.

67

In recent years, doubt has been expressed as to whether the so-called median palatine cyst is an entity or whether cysts in that region are merely posterior extensions of nasopalatine duct cysts. This point is discussed again later. Since 1968 we have therefore reported all developmental midline cysts of the maxilla as nasopalatine duct cysts.

Clinical Features

Frequency

Eighty-nine of the 750 jaw cysts accessioned in the Department have been nasopalatine duct cysts (11·9 per cent). These include the cysts which were originally diagnosed as median palatine cysts and those which were predominantly in the soft tissues and were called cysts of the palatine papilla. Some indication of the frequency of nasopalatine duct cysts in the general population may be determined from the fact that Killey and Kay (1972) reported finding two specimens with cysts in a study of the incisive fossae in 2394 skulls.

Age

The age distribution of 73 of our cases is shown in *Fig.* 50. There was no case in the first decade and the majority occurred in the fourth, fifth and sixth decades.

Sex

In our material there is a higher incidence of nasopalatine duct cysts in males than females ($P < 0.2$ per cent) and this sex predilection appears to be more marked in Blacks than in Whites although the difference is not statistically significant ($P > 10$ per cent). In a series of 89 patients, 70 were males (79 per cent) and 19 were females (21 per cent). This is a male : female ratio of 3·7 : 1. Of these, 38 were Black males and 7 Black females (5·4 : 1); 32 were White males and 12 were White females (2·7 : 1) (*Table* 6). Killey and Kay (1972) also recorded a male preponderance, but in the series of Abrams et al. (1963), there was an equal sex incidence.

In all, Blacks and Whites were equally involved.

Table 6.

SEX DISTRIBUTION OF BLACK AND WHITE PATIENTS WITH NASOPALATINE DUCT CYSTS

	Male	Female	Total	M : F ratio
Black	38	7	45	5·4 : 1
White	32	12	44	2·7 : 1
Total	70 (79%)	19 (21%)	89	3·7 : 1
W : B ratio	1 : 1·2	1 : 0·6	1 : 1	

Pa xxxxxx xxx xxxxxxxx xxxxxxxx xxxx xxxx xxx xxxxxxxxx xxxxxxxxxx xx xxxxxxxxxxx xxxx xxxxxx xxx xxxxxx xxxxx xx xxxxxx

Clinical Presentation

The most common symptom is swelling, usually in the anterior region of the midline of palate (*Figs.* 51 and 52). Swelling also occurs in the midline on the labial aspect of the alveolar ridge (*Fig.* 53) and in some cases 'through and through' fluctuation may be elicited between the labial and palatal swellings. It is when midline

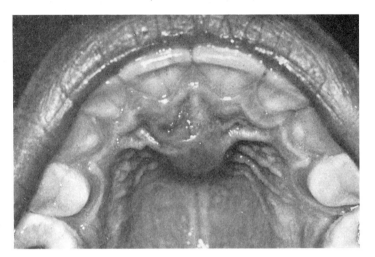

Fig. 51. Small nasopalatine duct cyst. (*Courtesy of Professor J. J. Pindborg.*)

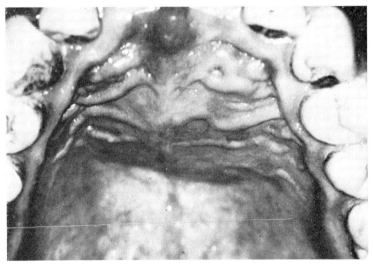

Fig. 52. Large nasopalatine duct cyst.

swellings of the palate occur further posteriorly that diagnoses of median palatine cysts tend to be made. In a number of our cases, the swelling has been associated with pain and discharge, but sometimes discharge is the only complaint and in a few cases pain is the only symptom. Various combinations of swelling, discharge and pain may occur. The discharge may be mucoid, in which case the patients sometimes describe a salty taste, or it may be purulent and patients complain of a foul taste. In patients with cysts of the palatine papilla, there may be a history of recurrent swellings which periodically discharge and then 'go down'.

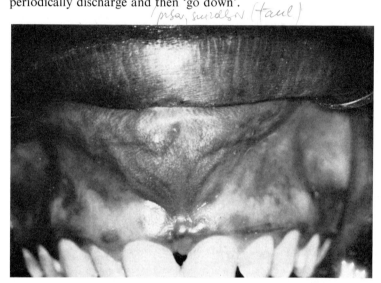

Fig. 53. Nasopalatine duct cyst producing a midline swelling of the labial aspect of the alveolar ridge.

In general, symptoms are not severe and patients often disregard them for many years. They may also be completely symptomless and be discovered fortuitously by the dentist during routine radiological examination and occasionally the presence of a cyst may become apparent after dentures are placed.

In establishing a diagnosis of nasopalatine duct cyst it is important to attempt to exclude the possibility of a periapical lesion by testing the pulp vitality of the incisor teeth.

Radiological Features

The nasopalatine duct cyst occurs in the incisive canal and it may be difficult to decide whether a radiolucency in that area is a cyst or a large incisive fossa. In attempting to distinguish between the two, the study done by Roper-Hall (1938) is frequently quoted. In an

70

investigation of 2162 skulls selected at random from a series of over 6000, he found that the incisive fossae of 2154 were absent or small. Five were of medium size, 1 was enlarged but shallow and 2 were large and cystic. The shapes of the fossae were round, oval, diamond or triangular and sometimes were funnel-shaped. Their antero-posterior measurement was usually greater than the width although the average measurements were 3 mm wide, 3 mm anteroposteriorly

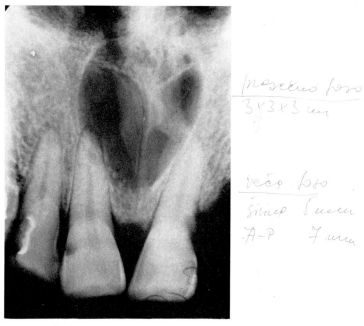

Fig. 54. Radiograph of a nasopalatine duct cyst. The lamina dura of the tooth on the left is intact although the apex appears to be in the cyst.

and 2–3 mm high. The largest fossa which was at all frequent was 5 mm wide and 7 mm anteroposteriorly. Of the 7 which were larger than this, 4 were 6 mm wide and 8 mm anteroposteriorly, and one was 6 mm wide and 10 mm anteroposteriorly. The two cavities which were large and cystic were 7 mm × 15 mm and 7 mm × 14 mm respectively. Roper-Hall concluded that any radiograph of the fossa which shows a shadow less than 6 mm wide may be considered to be within normal limits, provided the patients have no other symptoms. Similar observations made by Killey and Kay (1972) on 2394 fossae confirmed Roper-Hall's views.

Incisive canal cysts are found in the midline of the palate, above or between the roots of the central incisor teeth (*Fig.* 54). In the latter case, the incisor roots may diverge. Some cysts may appear heart-shaped either because they become notched by the nasal septum during their expansion, or because the nasal spine is superimposed on the radiolucent area, or if there are bilateral cysts. Cysts may develop bilaterally in both Stenson canals and in some instances the radiolucency may be seen laterally if a single cyst develops in one of the major lateral canals of Stenson (Stafne, 1969). Very large cysts extend posteriorly and superiorly and it is these which give rise to the diagnosis of median palatine cyst (*Fig.* 55). The margins of nasopalatine duct cysts are well-corticated unless they become infected.

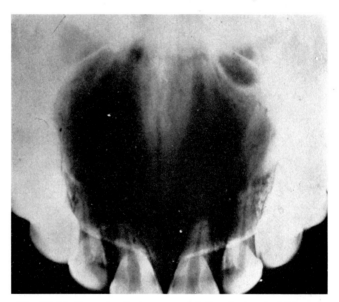

Fig. 55. Radiograph of a large nasopalatine duct cyst which may give rise to a diagnosis of median palatine cyst.

If on a dental radiograph the radiolucent area appears to be related to the apex of an incisor tooth, an occlusal view will usually demonstrate that the cyst and the apex are separated. In addition to the demonstration of pulp vitality, it may also be possible to see an intact lamina dura around the tooth apices (*Fig.* 54).

Pathogenesis
Nasopalatine duct cysts are thought to arise from the nasopalatine ducts in the incisive canal, but the aetiological factors associated with their formation and their pathogenesis are largely speculative.

72

In lower animals, the nasopalatine ducts are concerned in some way with the sense of smell. In man, vestigial remnants of this primitive organ of smell may be found in the incisive canals in the form of epithelial-lined ducts, epithelial cords, epithelial rests or combinations of these. Epithelial rests may show central degeneration. The frequency with which a continuous patent nasopalatine duct between the nasal and oral cavities occurs in man is uncertain as various authors have reported different findings. These are summarized by Abrams et al. (1963) who carried out similar studies on 24 fetuses. In none of these was there either a continuous patent duct or epithelial cords. In no instance did they find a patent oral opening of a nasopalatine duct, although 9 patent nasal openings were identified. Sixteen fetuses had portions of naso-palatine duct with central lumina and 3 of these had an appearance suggestive of cystic degeneration. In their investigation the ducts were lined most frequently by squamous epithelium (82 per cent of cases) and most of these were in the oral and middle thirds of the incisive canals. A primitive or cuboidal lining was present in 41 per cent of cases, and these were predominantly in the nasal third. Although squamous epithelium lined some nasopalatine ducts in the nasal third of the canal, in no case was pseudostratified columnar epithelium found in the oral third.

The vomer-nasal organs of Jacobson are sometimes mentioned as a possible source of cysts in the incisive canal but this is most unlikely. They are bilateral structures which lie at the base of the nasal septum just above the nasal extremity of the incisive canals. They are believed to be associated with the nasopalatine ducts as olfactory organs in many animals, and have been demonstrated in human embryos (Abrams et al., 1963).

As far as aetiology is concerned, it has been suggested that trauma or bacterial infection could stimulate the nasopalatine duct remnants to proliferate. There is, however, very little evidence to support such hypotheses. On the contrary, a number of factors tend to exclude these possibilities. If trauma to the area during mastication is the cause, why are the cysts found so infrequently when such trauma is very common? Why are the cysts so much more frequent in males than females? Some nasopalatine duct cysts, particularly those higher up in the canal away from the mouth, are relatively free of inflammatory infiltrate. Nor does one see arcading of proliferating stratified squamous epithelium as in inflamed radicular cysts. These latter two points do not of course definitely exclude the possibility of an inflammatory origin, as the inflammatory process could have subsided before the cyst was removed. They do, however, suggest that more evidence is required to support such a theory of onset. The fact that there may be an intense

73

inflammatory infiltrate in the walls of cysts of the palatine papilla is not really adequate evidence to support an inflammatory origin, as cysts of this region are more than likely to be traumatized and thereby show a secondary inflammatory infiltrate.

The fact that mucous glands develop in association with naso-palatine ducts and are sometimes seen in the walls of the cysts has led to the suggestion that the cysts might be caused by secretion of mucin from the glands into the duct lumina, particularly when the duct is blocked. Factors against such an origin are that only very infrequently have connections between the mucous glands and the duct lumina been demonstrated and that the secretory pressure that would exist is unlikely to be adequate to produce bone resorption and form an intraosseous cyst.

Main (1970a) has postulated that nasopalatine duct cysts, like primordial cysts, develop spontaneously. Although there is no proof for such an hypothesis, the concept is in accord with some of the facts. Firstly, there is the observation that small cystic dilatations of portions of the nasopalatine ducts are occasionally seen in fetal material. It would explain the absence of inflammatory cell infiltra-tions from so many cases and also the relative infrequency of the cysts in relation to the frequency of trauma in the nasopalatine area. Main (1970a) has shown that nasopalatine duct cysts show a lesser tendency than primordial cysts for epithelial proliferation, which partly explains their slow growth and moderate size. Main (1970b) believed that fluid accumulation is likely to be responsible for the enlargement of nasopalatine duct cysts but what leads to the initial collection of fluid in the cyst cavity is uncertain. Osmotic attraction of serum through normal capillary walls may occur and in the absence of drainage of this fluid (Toller, 1966b) the hydrostatic pressure would increase. Osmotically active particles are supplied by the breakdown of cells shed into the cyst cavity.

The mechanism which might initially trigger the spontaneous development of nasopalatine duct cysts, if this is indeed what happens, has yet to be identified. It seems to me possible that the occurrence of these cysts, as with other jaw cysts, may have some genetic determinant.

Histological Features (Figs. 56, 57, 58 and Table 7)

The epithelial linings of nasopalatine duct cysts are extremely variable. Stratified squamous, pseudostratified columnar, cuboidal, columnar, or primitive flat epithelium may be seen, individually or in combination. Goblet cells may be found in pseudostratified columnar epithelial linings, and cilia, although most frequently

74

seen on the surface of pseudostratified columnar epithelia, may also be present in association with columnar and, very rarely, with cuboidal epithelium.

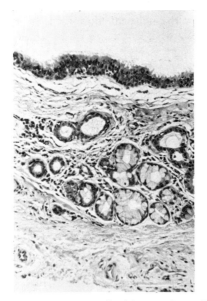

Fig. 56. Nasopalatine duct cyst lined by pseudostratified ciliated columnar epithelium. Mucous glands are present in the wall. HE; ×125.

Stratified squamous epithelium is found more frequently than any other, followed by pseudostratified columnar. In our own series of 86 cases, 67 (78 per cent) were lined by stratified squamous epithelium; 33 entirely, whereas 22 were lined in part by pseudostratified ciliated columnar epithelium. In the series, 39 cysts (45 per cent) contained pseudostratified ciliated columnar epithelium in part of their linings, but only 7 were lined entirely in this way. Four cysts were lined in part by simple columnar and 18 by simple cuboidal epithelium. One was lined entirely by cuboidal epithelium. These distributions are very similar to those of Abrams et al. (1963). Although it is frequently stated that cysts lined by respiratory epithelium originate from nasopalatine duct adjacent to the nasal cavity, whereas those lined by stratified squamous epithelium develop from the lower portion of the duct, this should not be regarded as a rule. For one thing, cysts of the palatine papilla may be lined by pseudostratified ciliated columnar epithelium, and for another, it is rare to find a nasopalatine duct cyst lined entirely by one variety of epithelium. Furthermore, except for cysts of the palatine papilla, it

75

is rare for a surgeon to state in his biopsy request what the anatomical level of any particular nasopalatine duct cyst was, so that it is not really possible to correlate position with histology. The fact that the majority of cyst linings have a combination of epithelial varieties is suggestive of their origin from pluripotential epithelium but the possibility that metaplasia occurs must also be considered.

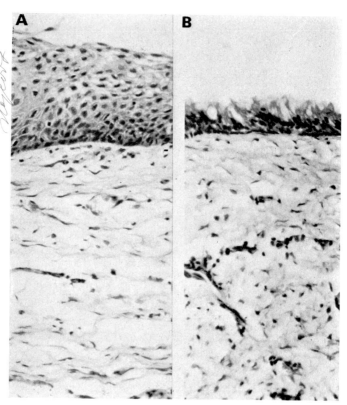

Fig. 57. Different areas in the nasopalatine duct cyst illustrated in *Fig.* 56. Part is lined by stratified squamous epithelium (A) and part by pseudostratified ciliated columnar epithelium (B). HE; ×225.

A valuable diagnostic feature of nasopalatine duct cysts is the presence of nerves and blood vessels in the fibrous capsule (*Fig.* 58). Abrams et al. (1963) showed that moderate-sized nerves were present in 88 per cent of their series and in the remaining 12 per cent nerves were present, although few and small. In 87 per cent of their cases, muscular arteries and numerous small veins were present. Our own observations support the frequency with which these features are found. In our series, prominent neurovascular bundles were found in 45 per cent of cases and large muscular arteries in 72 per cent. The explanation for this phenomenon is that the long sphenopalatine nerve and vessels which pass through the incisive canal are either included in the cyst wall or are removed with the cyst in the course of surgical enucleation.

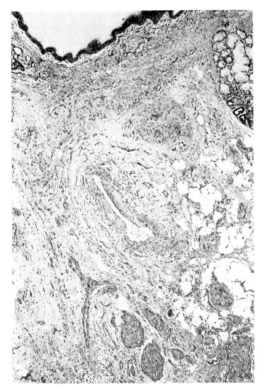

Fig. 58. Neurovascular bundle in the wall of a nasopalatine duct cyst. HE; ×40.

Small foci of mucous glands (*Fig.* 56) were found in the fibrous capsules of approximately one-third of cases in the series of Abrams et al. (1963), but in only 7 per cent of our own. As the foci are small, it is probable that their frequency would be higher if biopsy material were more extensively sampled. It has been suggested that the presence of mucous glands in a cyst wall is strong evidence in favour of the diagnosis of nasopalatine duct cyst, but I have seen them in an undoubted nasolabial cyst (*see Fig.* 65, p. 90).

77

bilateralus cyst

One patient in our series had bilateral cysts and in 19 cases (22 per cent) nasopalatine ducts or their remnants were present in the main cyst wall. In the study of Abrams et al. (1963), epithelial cell rests were found in the walls of 22 of 61 cysts (36 per cent).

Table 7.
HISTOLOGICAL FEATURES IN 86 NASOPALATINE DUCT CYSTS

		Numbers	Percentage
Epithelium			
Stratified squamous		67	78
entirely	33		
partly pseudostratified			
ciliated columnar	22		
partly cuboidal	10		
partly columnar	2		
Pseudostratified ciliated columnar		39	45
entirely	7		
partly squamous	22		
partly cuboidal	8		
partly columnar	2		
Fibrous cyst wall			
Neurovascular bundle		39	45
Large muscular-walled vessels		62	72
Mucous glands		6	7
Cartilage		6	7
Inflammatory infiltrate			
absent		21	24
mild		39	45
moderate		17	20
severe		9	11

6

otvore hyaline hmienica

As far as evidence of inflammation is concerned, we found that 21 of our cases (24 per cent) were relatively free of inflammatory cell infiltrate. In 39 (45 per cent) there was a mild chronic inflammatory cell infiltrate. In 17 (20 per cent) the chronic inflammatory process was graded as moderate and in 9 (11 per cent) as severe. In 2 cases there was a superimposed acute inflammatory cell infiltrate.

Small islands of hyaline cartilage may very rarely be seen in the cyst walls. They were present in 6 of our cases (7 per cent) and Abrams et al. (1963) found cartilage in all 4 of their palatine papilla cysts. These authors pointed out that unlike the incisive canal and surrounding palatal bone, the palatine papilla normally possessed a small accumulation of cartilage in its anterior aspect.

Treatment

Nasopalatine duct cysts are treated by surgical enucleation. A palatal flap is reflected after an incision along the gingival margins of the teeth. After severing the neurovascular bundle, the cyst is exposed, if necessary by the removal of bone. The cyst is then carefully dissected from the bony canal. Blood clot is allowed to fill the cavity and the flap is then sutured (Killey and Kay, 1972). Recurrences have not been reported.

CHAPTER 9

THE SO-CALLED MEDIAN PALATINE, MEDIAN ALVEOLAR, MEDIAN MANDIBULAR AND GLOBULOMAXILLARY CYSTS

MEDIAN PALATINE AND MEDIAN ALVEOLAR CYSTS

IN recent years, the existence of separate entities of median palatine and median alveolar cyst has been questioned and they have been excluded from the World Health Organization Classification (Pindborg and Kramer, 1971). Previously it was thought that these cysts developed from epithelium entrapped in the process of fusion of embryonic processes, whereas it is now felt that they represent posterior extension of an incisive canal cyst in the case of median palatine cyst, and anterior extension in the case of median alveolar cyst.

Reference has been made elsewhere (Chapter 3) to the presence of cysts along the midpalatal raphe which arise from epithelial inclusions at the line of fusion of the palatal folds and the nasal processes. After birth the epithelial inclusions usually atrophy and become resorbed, but some may produce keratin-containing microcysts (*Fig.* 21, p. 29) which extend to the surface and rupture during the first few months after birth. These are not, however, what are usually referred to as median palatine or median posterior palatine cysts, which are described as intrabony cysts in the midline of the palate. If a median posterior palatine cyst indeed exists it would be necessary to postulate its origin as being by enlargement of a midpalatine raphe cyst, or from epithelial inclusions in the region (Courage et al., 1974). The contingency of this occurring must be remote. The midpalatine raphe cysts and the epithelial inclusions lie close to the palatal epithelium. It seems unlikely that a median palatine cyst could develop in this site and produce extensive bone resorption without forming a large palatal swelling at a very much earlier stage of its natural history.

I have re-examined the histological sections of 15 cases which were diagnosed as median palatine cysts in our department until 1968 when we stopped making this diagnosis. Six of these were lined exclusively by stratified squamous epithelium while the remaining 9 were lined in part by pseudostratified ciliated columnar, cuboidal or columnar epithelium. Of the 6 lined exclusively by stratified squamous epithelium, 3 contained neurovascular bundles in the wall and another 2 contained large muscular blood vessels. Two of this group also showed remnants of nasopalatine ducts in their walls. There was no evidence of mucous glands in the walls of any of the 15 cases. These histological features would be consistent with a diagnosis of a nasopalatine duct cyst.

As far as the median alveolar cyst of the maxilla is concerned, Sicher (1962) is convinced that there is no embryological basis for assuming that it develops from epithelium enclaved at the site of fusion between the right and left globular processes. 'Such a fusion', says Sicher, 'simply does not occur.'

MEDIAN MANDIBULAR CYST

Very occasionally, a cyst occurs in the midline of the mandible. It produces a well-defined round or ovoid or irregular radiolucent area and may separate the roots of the lower incisor teeth (*Fig.* 59).

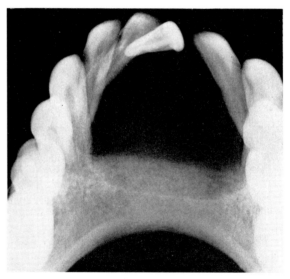

Fig. 59. A so-called median mandibular cyst which proved to be a primordial cyst on histological examination.

In some of the reported cases, the associated teeth have given non-vital pulp responses (Olech, 1957: Case 2; Albers, 1973) and in others they have all been vital (Olech, 1957: Case 1; Meyer, 1957; Lucchesi and Topazian, 1961; Blair and Wadsworth, 1968; Killey and Kay, 1972; Buchner and Ramon, 1974).

The presence of a cyst in the midline of the mandible associated with vital teeth tempted some workers to propose its origin from epithelial inclusions trapped in the area during embryonic development. This concept is, however, not tenable as the mandible forms in the mandibular process which develops as a single unit. As no fusion takes place between ectodermal processes it is not possible to postulate that epithelial entrapment occurs.

Those cysts associated with teeth which have non-vital pulps are very likely to be radicular, and when these are lined by ciliated pseudostratified columnar epithelium it may very possibly be the result of secretory metaplasia. Olech's Case 1 and Meyer's case show histological features which resemble but are not identical to those of primordial cysts. The two cases reported by Buchner and Ramon appear to be primordial cysts. The published photomicrographs of the cases reported by Lucchesi and Topazian and by Blair and Wadsworth show a thin epithelial lining resembling reduced enamel epithelium and may possibly be lateral periodontal cysts. Killey and Kay's case was a simple bone cyst.

There is little evidence, therefore, to indicate that the median mandibular cyst is an entity.

GLOBULOMAXILLARY CYST

The globulomaxillary cyst has traditionally been described as a fissural cyst found within the bone between the maxillary lateral incisor and canine teeth. Radiologically it is a well-defined radiolucency which frequently causes the roots of the adjacent teeth to diverge (*Fig.* 60). While there can be no doubt that cysts do occur in this region and that the pulps of the adjacent teeth may give positive vitality responses, there is now a considerable body of opinion against the idea that they are fissural cysts. The evidence against their being fissural cysts is in fact more substantial than the evidence in favour.

The first description of the globulomaxillary cyst has been ascribed to Thoma (1937), but I have not been able to verify this. It was believed for many years that they were fissural cysts arising from non-odontogenic epithelium included at the site of fusion of the globular process of the medial (frontonasal) process, and the maxillary process. A variation of this concept was proposed by Ferenczy (1958) who considered that these cysts form at the junction of the premaxilla and maxilla, and that they should be called premaxillary-maxillary cysts. In 1962, Sicher seriously questioned the traditional theory of origin of globulomaxillary cysts, stating that on embryological grounds such an explanation was impossible. He believed that cysts in that region were probably primordial.

82

Embryologists have pointed out (Arey, 1965) that the surface bulges seen in the nasomaxillary complex of the embryo and which are called 'facial processes' are not in fact prolongations with free ends which meet in the nasal region. Other than at the median palatal raphe there is no ectoderm-to-ectoderm contact which requires dissolution of the ectodermal surfaces prior to fusion and there is therefore no possibility of enclavement of ectodermal residues. The facial processes are in fact merely elevations or ridges

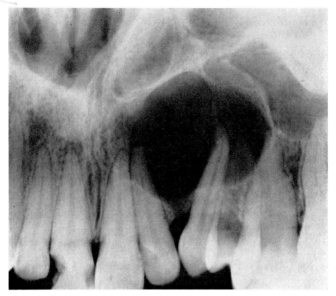

Fig. 60. Status X radiograph of a cyst in the 'globulomaxillary' region. Histologically this was a primordial cyst.

which correspond to centres of growth in the underlying mesenchyme. These are covered by a continuous sheet of folded epithelium. As these growth centres proliferate and develop, the surface furrows between them become more shallow and eventually smooth out.

A critical study of the whole question of globulomaxillary cysts was reported by Christ (1970). In a survey of the literature over the 50-year period 1920–69, he found very few cases which fulfilled the criteria for acceptance, namely, a radiograph of the lesion, positive vitality of adjacent teeth, and tissue sections or photomicrographs of the histological material. He pointed out that his literature review revealed that a wide variety of other lesions present clinically and radiologically as globulomaxillary cysts. These included adenomatoid odontogenic tumours, myxoma and haemorrhagic bone

83

cyst. Many cases were reported in the literature as globulomaxillary cysts despite the fact that there were non-vital or absent lateral incisors or canines.

He also reviewed 27 cases from his own departmental records and found that only 3 satisfied the criteria for inclusion in his study. Histologically, two of these appeared to be primordial cysts and the other was thought to be of odontogenic origin. He suggested, therefore, that the globulomaxillary cyst is in fact an odontogenic cyst and that its clinical and radiological appearances may fit the diagnosis of lateral periodontal, lateral dentigerous and primordial cyst.

Zegarelli and Zegarelli (1973) emphasized also that the globulomaxillary region is a potential site for a wide range of pathologic entities and a definitive diagnosis should not be made before histopathological examination.

A review of 17 of our own cases accessioned as globulomaxillary cysts tends to support Christ's views. Only 6 of them showed any semblance of respiratory epithelium. Two of the cases had the classic histological features of primordial cysts; 4 were associated with missing or root-treated teeth; 4 had histological features very much like those seen in lateral periodontal cysts; and in 5 the clinical information was quite inadequate for a definitive diagnosis. There remained 2 possible cases, and even in these the clinical information was equivocal and the respiratory epithelium in the cyst linings could be explained on the basis of metaplasia.

A different point of view has however been put forward by Little and Jakobsen (1973). They quoted Patten (1961) in support of their belief that processes which join by merging may still entrap epithelium between them if mesenchymal growth is retarded below the groove that separates them. They believed too that the 'epithelial wall' which forms by fusion of the medial nasal process and the maxillary process at the inferior margin of the nasal pit is another potential source of epithelial remnants, despite the fact that these have not been found in studies of normal fetal tissues. Although agreeing that the globular process is not involved, they believed that a developmental cyst could arise from these epithelial residues. They suggested that cysts in this region of the maxilla may therefore be of either odontogenic or non-odontogenic epithelial origin.

My own conclusions are, however, that the following facts tend to indicate that the cysts found in the 'globulomaxillary' area are not fissural cysts and are probably of odontogenic origin.

1. Even when the diagnosis of globulomaxillary cyst is made uncritically, it is made very rarely.

2. Most embryologists deny the possibility of ectodermal inclusions other than in the midpalatine raphe and the nasolacrimal rod,

and there is no direct evidence from studies of fetal tissues to support the view of some that epithelial inclusions do occur in the globulo-maxillary area.

3. Histologically, a number of them have the features of primordial cysts.

4. Clinically, radiologically and histologically, a number of them fulfil the criteria for the diagnosis of lateral periodontal cyst.

5. A cyst in that area may be a radicular cyst associated with the lateral or canine teeth; and when teeth are missing in the area, it may be a residual radicular cyst.

DD: — odontogenic tumor
— myxoma
— neurofibrous histans cyst

CHAPTER 10

NASOLABIAL (NASOALVEOLAR) CYST

THE nasolabial cyst occurs outside the bone in the nasolabial folds below the alae nasi. It is traditionally regarded as a jaw cyst although strictly speaking it should be classified as a soft-tissue cyst.

Clinical Features

Frequency

Nasolabial cysts are rare lesions and our own material consists of only 5 examples seen in 15 years. Roed-Petersen (1969), in an extensive review of the literature, found information relating to 155 patients with nasolabial cysts and has done a statistical analysis of the combined data of 111 of these patients plus 5 of his own cases. These data are presented below.

Age

There is a wide age distribution ranging from 12 to 75 years, with most of the cases occurring in the third to the sixth decades (*Fig.* 61).

Sex

There is a considerable preponderance of females with nasolabial cysts. In Roed-Petersen's review, of 116 patients 90 were female (78 per cent) and 26 male (22 per cent), a female : male ratio of 3·5 : 1. This difference is statistically significant ($P<0·001$).

Clinical Presentation

The most frequent symptom is swelling and very often this is the only complaint. Sometimes the patients complain of pain and difficulty in nasal breathing. In some cases, difficulty with an upper denture has drawn attention to the problem, and occasionally the cysts are diagnosed fortuitously during routine examination. In most cases the cysts are unilateral, but in the Roed-Petersen study 13 (11·2 per cent) patients had bilateral lesions.

The cysts grow slowly, producing a swelling of the lip. They fill out the nasolabial fold and may lift the ala nasi, distort the nostril and produce a swelling of the floor of the nose. Intraorally they form a bulge in the labial sulcus (*Fig.* 62). The cysts are fluctuant and, on bimanual palpation, fluctuation may be elicited between the swelling on the floor of the nose and that in the labial sulcus. Infected cysts may discharge into the nose.

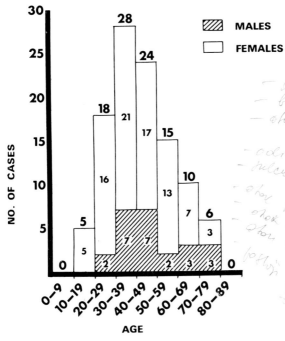

Fig. 61. Age distribution of 106 patients with nasolabial cysts. (*After Roed-Petersen, 1969.*)

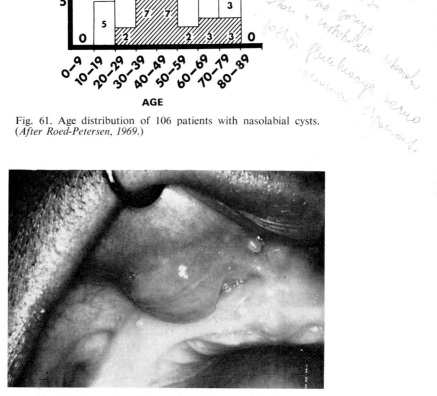

Fig. 62. Intraoral swelling produced by a nasolabial cyst.

87

Radiological Features

A detailed description of the radiological features has been provided by Seward (1962). He pointed out that there is a localized increased radiolucency of the alveolar process above the apices of the incisor teeth. This radiolucency results from a depression on the labial surface of the maxilla which may be detectable in a tangential view. When the depression extends to the lateral margin of the anterior bony aperture of the nose there is resorption of the lower part of the nasal notch. The inferior margin of the anterior bony aperture of the nose is distorted by the lesion. As a result, standard occlusal radiographs show a pronounced posterior convexity in one half of the bracket-shaped radio-opaque line which forms the bony border of the nasal aperture, instead of the usual double curve (*Fig.* 63).

The cyst may be aspirated and a radio-opaque liquid introduced, after which it may be viewed in tangential and postero-anterior views of the jaws or in vertex occlusal views (*Fig.* 64). It is normally a spherical or kidney-shaped lesion lying against the inferior and lateral borders of the anterior bony aperture of the nose, extending from the midline to the canine fossa.

Pathogenesis

The pathogenesis of the nasolabial cyst is unresolved. The traditional concept, as described in many textbooks, is that the nasolabial cyst is the soft-tissue equivalent of the globulomaxillary cyst. It has therefore been suggested that it arises from epithelium enclaved at the site of fusion of the globular, lateral nasal and maxillary processes. This concept, however, is not really tenable as the embryologic basis for it has been seriously disputed (*see* discussion in section on globulomaxillary cysts, Chapter 9). Fløe Møller and Philipsen (1958), Seward (1962) and Roed-Petersen (1969) have reviewed the various hypotheses proposed to explain the origin of nasolabial cysts, and one of the suggestions is that they develop from the lower anterior part of the nasolacrimal duct. When the margins of the lateral nasal and maxillary bulges coalesce, the ectoderm along the boundary between them gives rise to a solid cellular rod which at first develops as a linear surface elevation, the nasolacrimal ridge, and then sinks into the mesenchyme. Its caudal end proliferates to connect with the caudal part of the lateral nasal wall while its cranial extremity later connects with the developing conjunctival sac. This solid rod then becomes canalized to form the nasolacrimal duct (Warwick and Williams, 1973). The location of nasolabial cysts is such that they could conceivably develop from remnants of the embryonic nasolacrimal rod or duct, if not from the lower anterior portion of the mature duct. The mature nasolacrimal duct is lined by pseudostratified columnar epithelium and this is

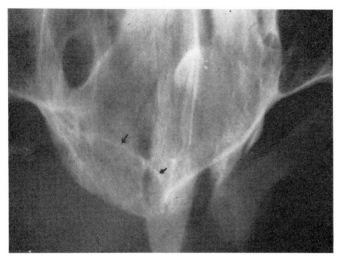

Fig. 63. Standard occlusal view of a patient with a nasolabial cyst. There is posterior bulging of the right side of the bracket shaped line, indicated by arrows. (*Courtesy of Professor G. R. Seward and the Editor*, The Dental Practitioner. *Previously published* (*1962*) Dent. Pract. **12**, 154–161.)

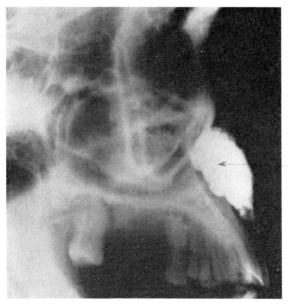

Fig. 64. Nasolabial cyst demonstrated radiologically by aspiration of its fluid contents and injection of a radio-opaque fluid.

the type of epithelium usually found lining nasolabial cysts. Further embryological studies on the nasolacrimal duct could be of value in solving this problem.

Whatever the cells of origin of nasolabial cysts, they do seem to be of developmental origin, and this is supported by the frequent occurrence of bilateral examples.

Histological Features

The 5 examples in our collection are all lined by non-ciliated pseudostratified columnar epithelium (*Fig.* 65). Goblet cells, varying

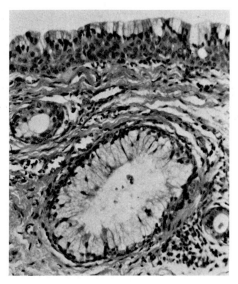

Fig. 65. Nasolabial cyst. It is lined by pseudostratified columnar epithelium containing many goblet cells. In the example illustrated here, mucous glands are present in the wall. HE; ×150.

in number from very few to very many, were seen in 4 of them. In one case there were small, localized areas of squamous metaplasia. In 2 cases the surface layers of the epithelial lining were eroded leaving a single layer of flat epithelium on the luminal surface and in some parts of these specimens the entire epithelial thickness was eroded leaving discontinuities.

The fibrous cysts walls were relatively acellular and either loosely or densely collagenous. Two of the walls which consisted of loose connective tissue were very haemorrhagic. One cyst wall was fairly intensely infiltrated with chronic inflammatory cells while the others were relatively uninflamed. Mucous glands lay close to the epithelial cyst lining in one instance.

In Roed-Petersen's review, 64 cases which had been evaluated histologically were summarized. Pseudostratified columnar epithelium was the only type of lining in 26 cases (41 per cent). In 9, pseudostratified columnar epithelium was present in association with stratified squamous epithelium, and in 15 with cuboidal epithelium. Seven cases contained stratified squamous and cuboidal epithelium, 4 contained only cuboidal epithelium and 3 were lined by pseudostratified columnar, stratified squamous and cuboidal epithelium. In all, 53 of the cases (83 per cent) were lined wholly or in part by pseudostratified columnar epithelium. Goblet cells were present in 33 cysts and ciliated cells in 22.

Treatment

Nasolabial cysts are treated by surgical excision through an intraoral approach. A mucoperiosteal flap is reflected and the cyst is separated from the surrounding tissues by blunt dissection. There is no tendency to recurrence, but the operation is often complicated by perforation of the nasal mucosa, particularly if the cyst has previously discharged into the nose.

91

CHAPTER 11

RADICULAR CYST

A RADICULAR cyst is one which arises from the epithelial residues in the periodontal ligament as a result of inflammation. The inflammation usually follows the death of the dental pulp and cysts arising in this way are found most commonly at the apices of the involved

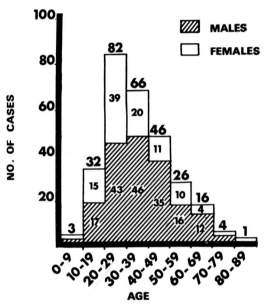

Fig. 66. Age distribution of 276 South African patients with radicular cysts.

teeth. They may however also be found on the lateral aspects of the roots in relation to lateral accessory root canals. Less commonly, inflammatory cysts may occur towards the cervical margin of the lateral aspect of a root as a consequence of an inflammatory process in a periodontal pocket. The latter lesion is perhaps best referred to as an inflammatory periodontal cyst or inflammatory collateral cyst (Main, 1970a, b) to distinguish it from radicular cysts resulting from pulp death, and from the lateral periodontal cyst which is of developmental origin. Quite often a radicular cyst remains behind in the jaws after removal of the offending tooth and this is referred to as a residual cyst.

92

Clinical Features

Frequency

Radicular and residual cysts are by far the most common cystic lesions in the jaws, comprising 433 (57·7 per cent) of 750 jaw cysts in our series (*see Table* 1, p. 6). This is a somewhat lower frequency than the figure of 67 per cent in the series of Killey and Kay (1972).

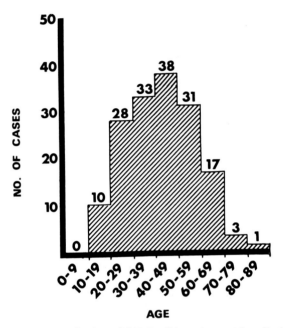

Fig. 67. Age distribution of 161 English patients with radicular cysts.

Age

The age distribution of 276 patients in our series is shown in *Fig. 66*. Very few cases are seen in the first decade, after which there is a fairly steep rise, with a peak incidence in the third decade. There are large numbers of cases in the fourth and fifth decades, after which there is a gradual decline. The low incidence in the first decade has been shown in a number of studies and indicates that although dental caries is frequently found in children during the first decade, radicular cysts are not commonly found associated with deciduous teeth.

Interestingly, an age distribution analysis which I did some years ago of a group of English patients with radicular cysts (*Fig.* 67) suggests that the majority of these cysts tend to be found at a somewhat older age in the English than the South African group.

Statistically, the difference is significant at the 0·025 level (Chi² = 23·9; D.O.F. 11). This difference between the two populations may mean that the South African group are exposed to the relevant aetiological factor, mainly dental caries, at an earlier age than the English group.

Sex

Of 366 cases in our series, 231 (63 per cent) were in males and 135 (37 per cent) in females, a statistically significant difference ($P < 0·1$ per cent). This ratio of 1·7 : 1 is very similar to that reported by other workers. The lower incidence in females may be because they are less likely to neglect their teeth, particularly the maxillary anterior incisors, in which area a large proportion of radicular cysts occur. Males moreover are more likely to sustain trauma to their maxillary anterior teeth.

Race

In our sample White patients were involved more frequently than Black (1·7 : 1).

Site

The anatomical distribution of 789 cysts from a pooled sample of South African and English patients is shown in *Fig.* 68. They occur in all tooth-bearing areas of the jaws although about 60 per cent are found in the maxilla and 40 per cent in the mandible. There is a particularly high incidence in the maxillary anterior region (37 per cent) and there are a number of possible reasons for this. Maxillary incisors have in the past, perhaps more frequently than other teeth, had silicate restorations placed in them, with consequent high risk to their pulps. Then there is the high incidence of palatal invaginations in the maxillary lateral incisors and the frequency with which pulp death supervenes in these teeth; and thirdly, maxillary anterior teeth are probably more prone than others to traumatic injuries which lead to pulp death.

Clinical Presentation

Many radicular cysts are symptomless and are discovered when periapical radiographs are taken of teeth with non-vital pulps. Slowly enlarging swellings are often complained of. At first the enlargement is bony hard but as the cyst increases in size, the covering bone becomes very thin despite subperiosteal bone deposition and the swelling then exhibits 'springiness'. Only when the cyst has completely eroded the bone will there be fluctuation. In the maxilla there may be buccal or palatal enlargement whereas in the mandible it is usually labial or buccal and only rarely lingual.

94

Pain and infection are other clinical features of some radicular cysts. It is often said that radicular cysts are painless unless infected. Some patients with these lesions, however, complain of pain although no evidence of infection is found clinically and no evidence of acute inflammation is seen histologically after the cyst has been removed. Likewise, some patients have clinically infected and histologically inflamed cysts which are not painful (Shear, 1961a).

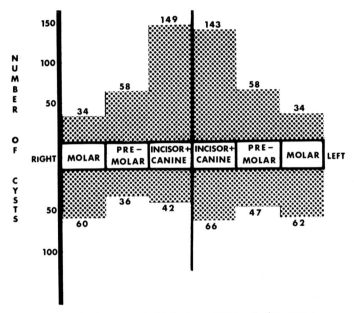

Fig. 68. Anatomical distribution of 789 radicular cysts.

A *sine qua non* for the diagnosis of a radicular cyst is the related presence of a tooth with a non-vital pulp. Occasionally, a sinus may lead from the cyst cavity to the oral mucosa.

Quite often, more than one radicular cyst may be found in a patient (Shear, 1961a; Stoelinga, 1973) and this has led a number of authors to believe that there are cyst-prone individuals who show a particular susceptibility to develop radicular cysts (Oehlers, 1970). This view is supported by the fact that radicular cysts are relatively rare in relation to the vast numbers of grossly carious teeth with dead pulps. It is possible that an immune mechanism may inhibit cyst formation in most individuals and that cyst-prone subjects have a defective immunological surveillance and suppression mechanism (Toller, 1970a).

Radiological Features

A number of studies have shown that it is difficult to differentiate radiologically between radicular cysts and apical granulomas. Mortensen et al. (1970) examined histological material of 396 periapical lesions with a diameter of 5 mm or more, which had been classified preoperatively as cysts or granulomas on radiological evidence. A correct preliminary diagnosis had been made in 81 per cent of 232 granulomas but in only 48 per cent of 164 cysts. They also showed that the relative number of granulomas decreases with increasing size of the lesion whereas there is an increase in the relative number of cysts. Nevertheless it is interesting to note that of all the lesions measuring 10–14 mm in radiographic diameter, there were almost as many granulomas as cysts; and that in their group of lesions measuring 15 mm or more, approximately one-third were granulomas. Moreover, a little over one-third of their lesions measuring 5–9 mm were cysts on histological examination.

These data certainly indicate that one cannot rely on the size of the lesion to establish a diagnosis. In addition, the large number of cysts which were incorrectly diagnosed as granulomas suggested to the authors that because of infection many cysts have a diffuse radiographic margin and therefore lack the circumscribed appearance usually ascribed to radicular cysts.

The classic description of the radiological appearance of radicular cysts is that they are round or ovoid radiolucencies surrounded by a narrow radio-opaque margin which extends from the lamina dura of the involved tooth (*Fig.* 69). In infected or rapidly enlarging cysts the radio-opaque margin may not be present. This can lead to diagnostic problems in the case of residual cysts. With a residual cyst, moreover, the differential diagnosis of primordial cyst must be considered. A radicular cyst on the lateral margin of a root in association with an accessory root canal must be differentiated from a lateral periodontal cyst. Root resorption is rare, but may occur.

Pathogenesis

It is convenient to consider the pathogenesis of radicular cysts in three phases: the phase of initiation, the phase of cyst formation and the phase of enlargement. The precise mechanisms involved in all phases are controversial. It is generally agreed that the epithelial linings of these cysts are derived from the epithelial cell rests of Malassez in the periodontal ligament. There is also no doubt that these cells may proliferate, and when they do so, either *in vivo*, or in tissue culture experiments, there are consistent morphological and histochemical changes (Ten Cate, 1972). The proliferating cells show a decrease in nucleo-cytoplasmic ratio, they utilize glycogen, synthesize neutral lipid and ribonucleic acid, and show an increased glucose-6-phosphate dehydrogenase activity but depressed succinic dehydrogenase activity. The latter two chemical changes indicate that the activated epithelial cells preferentially use the hexose–monophosphate shunt.

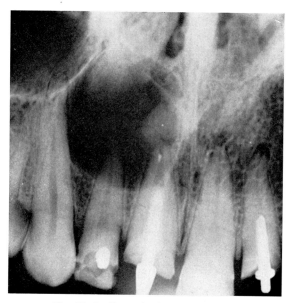

Fig. 69. Radiograph of a radicular cyst.

Precisely how these epithelial cells are stimulated to proliferate is not clear. It would seem that some product of a dead pulp may initiate the process and that at the same time it evokes an inflammatory reaction as there is evidence (Shear, 1963a) that proliferating odontogenic epithelium is associated with the presence of an acute inflammatory cell infiltration. A feature of this infiltrate is that the polymorphonuclear leucocytes are found in the proliferating epithelium (Shear, 1964), and it may be that the substance which initiates the epithelial proliferation exerts a direct effect on the epithelium itself and is also chemotactic to polymorphonuclear leucocytes.

There is also some evidence however that local changes in the supporting connective tissue may be responsible for activating the cell rests (Grupe et al., 1967) and that a decreased oxygen and increased carbon dioxide tension and a local reduction in pH produced in chronic inflammation may be the critical factors.

97

Proliferating epithelium has a characteristic histological appearance. The epithelium, in section, forms arcades and rings each encircling a core of vascular connective tissue. The reason for this appearance may be appreciated by considering the three-dimensional picture. When the epithelial cells proliferate, they do so in different planes, forming a mass rather than sheets or strands. Cores of vascular connective tissue extend into the epithelial mass from all directions and the resulting appearance in histological section is one of arcades and rings of epithelial cells surrounding these cores. This epithelial arcading is frequently seen in histological preparations of apical granulomas and radicular cysts (*Fig.* 70).

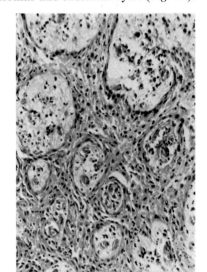

Fig. 70. Arcades and rings of epithelium in an apical granuloma. HE; ×125.

The next phase in the pathogenesis of a radicular cyst is the process by which a cavity comes to be lined by the proliferating odontogenic epithelium. Two possibilities are generally recognized and I believe in fact that both are feasible and both may operate independently of one another. One concept proposes that the epithelium proliferates and covers the bare connective tissue surface of an abscess cavity or a cavity which may occur as a result of connective tissue breakdown by proteolytic enzyme activity (Summers, 1974). The other, which probably occurs more frequently, postulates that a cyst cavity forms within a proliferating epithelial mass in an apical granuloma by degeneration and death of cells in the centre.

There is histological evidence for the latter hypothesis. The proliferating epithelial masses show considerable intercellular oedema. These intercellular accumulations of fluid coalesce to form microcysts containing epithelial and inflammatory cells (*Fig.* 71). The demonstration of high levels of acid phosphatase activity in the central cells of apical granulomas (Grupe et al., 1967) and in the exfoliating epithelial cells of radicular cysts (Lutz et al., 1965), and the fact that Summers (1972, 1974) found that weak proteolytic activity was present centrally within the proliferating epithelium of apical granulomas, suggest that these cells are undergoing autolysis.

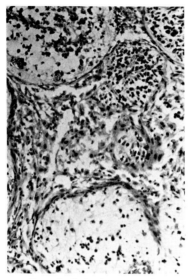

Fig. 71. Degeneration of cells in the centre of a mass of proliferating epithelium in an apical granuloma. Accumulations of intercellular fluid coalesce to form a microcyst. HE; × 50.

Moreover, ultrastructural examination of epithelial islands in experimentally induced granulomas shows evidence of death of the central cells (Ten Cate, 1972). Microcysts may increase in size by coalescence with adjacent microcysts and, once established, the cyst increases in size by accumulation of fluid within its cavity.

This third phase in the pathogenesis of radicular cysts is also controversial. Toller's experimental work provides evidence for the hypothesis that most cysts increase in size as a result of osmosis. He has shown (1970b) that the mean osmolality of the fluid from 21 apical and residual cysts was 290±14·93 milliosmoles compared with a mean serum osmolality of 279±4·68 milliosmoles. This difference is statistically significant at the 1 per cent level. Lytic products of the epithelial and inflammatory cells in the cyst cavity provide the greater numbers of smaller molecules which raise the osmotic pressure of the cyst fluid. Toller believed that the upper limit of permeability in most cysts is close to the molecular size of albumin, molecular weight 69 000, and that particles of larger size would find difficulty in diffusing across a cyst lining. Toller's *in vivo* dialysis experiments (1966b) using a radioactive crystalloid and a radioactive colloid showed that the diffusion rate of the crystalloid was fairly rapid in every case but that the colloid tended to be retained, whether subsequent histological examination revealed that the cyst wall was entirely lined by epithelium or not. This tended to confirm that cyst walls have the properties of a semipermeable membrane.

Electrophoretic studies (Toller, 1970a) demonstrated that radicular cyst fluids contain fewer, if any, of the larger protein molecules than the patients' own sera. Alpha-globulins were greatly diminished. Gamma-globulin varied greatly in quantity but in cysts which were not inflamed was present in small concentration. The small molecular sized albumin, and $beta_1$-globulin, were present in quantities comparable with serum but $beta_2$-globulin was usually absent. This suggested that these cyst fluids were simple dialysates from plasma through the cyst membranes which discriminate against the larger molecules.

Toller (1966b) also proposed the hypothesis that the contents of cyst cavities are subject to an osmotic imbalance with the surrounding tissues because of the absence of lymphatic drainage. He demonstrated this absence of lymphatic drainage by evacuating cyst cavities and refilling them with an aqueous solution of patent blue dye. At operation from 3 to 24 hours later, he was unable to detect any dye outside the cyst cavity. Neither the patients nor their urine were discoloured.

Main (1970b), however, felt that the retention of colloid in Toller's experiment may have resulted from a reduced internal hydrostatic pressure following aspiration of the fluid contents. He estimated the protein concentrations of cyst fluids by means of specific gravity and concluded that the radicular cyst fluid is essentially an inflammatory exudate. This view is supported by Skaug (1973) who confirmed that fluid from non-keratinizing jaw cysts contains high concentrations of protein.

In a later paper, Skaug (1974) commented on the question of permeability of cyst walls. He pointed out that the cyst capsule was not directly comparable to the biological membranes like capillary walls or cell membranes because of the many layers of cells of diverse function. These were the vascular endothelium, basement membranes, ground substance and cyst wall epithelium. The view that

100

the cyst wall functions as a simple semipermeable membrane is therefore probably an oversimplification. It may nevertheless still be preferable to use the term permeability in connection with the passage of substances into or away from the cyst cavity.

Skaug found that the concentration of non-immunoglobulin plasma proteins in cyst fluids was proportionate to their concentration in plasma and, as Toller did, that these were in inverse proportion to their molecular weights. The demonstration in cyst fluid of appreciable amounts of high molecular weight proteins suggested that the vascular permeability of cyst capsules was increased compared to the permeability of normal capillaries but there is nevertheless still a considerable restriction to free diffusion of plasma protein across the cyst capsule.

Toller (1948) showed that the internal hydrostatic pressures in 51 radicular cysts ranged from 56·6 to 95·0 cm water with a mean of 70·0 cm. This figure is higher than that of capillary blood pressure and as the cyst expands there is resorption of the surrounding bone.

Harris and Goldhaber (1973) have demonstrated that small fragments of vital cyst tissue produced resorption of mouse calvarium in tissue culture, whereas control tissue devitalized by rapid freezing and thawing failed to resorb bone. They postulated that intra-osseous cyst expansion is facilitated by local enzyme or hormone-induced bone resorption and suggested that the active principal is a prostaglandin. In a subsequent publication, Harris et al. (1973) were able to show that extracts of cyst did contain substantial amounts of prostaglandin-like material.

There do not appear to be data on the rate of radicular cyst growth although it has been estimated at approximately 5 mm in diameter annually (Livingston, 1927). They tend to expand progressively and if untreated may grow to a large size. The larger the cyst, however, the slower its relative increase in size.

Epithelial proliferation continues as long as there is an inflammatory stimulus, but probably plays very little, if any, part in the growth of the cyst. When the stimulus to epithelial proliferation ceases, a situation which often occurs in a residual cyst, the epithelium is able to differentiate to a certain extent (*Fig.* 72), although keratinization is very rare. Further increase in the capacity of the cyst cavity at this stage probably leads to thinning of the epithelial lining.

A model for the experimental production of radicular cysts would be of considerable value in elucidating some of the problems enunciated above. Some useful studies in this respect have been published by Binnie and Rowe (1974) and Valderhaug (1974). Binnie and Rowe studied 192 roots of immature pulpless teeth in 8 young beagle dogs. The pulps had been filled with various materials.

101

Epithelial cell rests were observed in 49 roots and proliferating epithelium in 14. Nine periapical cysts were found in 4 dogs. The authors noted considerable variation between different dogs and this may reinforce the concept of individual susceptibility to the development of radicular cysts. In one dog, only one root showed epithelium, but in another there was epithelium associated with 19 of the 24 roots examined and 4 of these had formed cysts. All

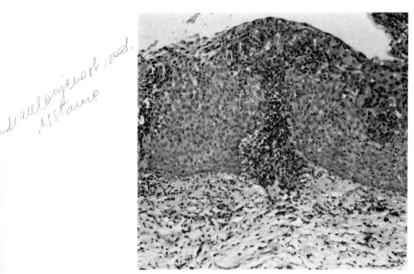

Fig. 72. Quiescent epithelium lining a radicular cyst. HE; ×90.

epithelial proliferations and cysts were associated with mild or severe periapical inflammation but their incidence was not related to the filling material used. An interesting feature of this study was the finding that epithelial remnants were present in only 37 per cent of specimens. If a similar situation obtains in humans, this alone may explain the existence of cyst-prone and non-cyst-prone individuals.

Valderhaug induced periapical inflammation in monkey primary teeth by removing the pulp tissue and leaving the root canals open to the oral cavity. About a third of the experimental teeth developed periapical abscesses, granulomas and cysts without communication with the oral cavity. Proliferating epithelium was not observed in association with abscess formation. Many of the granulomas, however, contained islands and strands of proliferating epithelial cells. Small periapical cysts developed in some animals after long observation periods and these were lined by stratified squamous epithelium. [3]H thymidine was incorporated into the epithelial

102

linings of the cysts and into the epithelium of the granulomas in inflamed areas. Uptake by epithelium could not be demonstrated at a certain distance from the inflammation nor on the control side.

Pathological Features

The gross specimens may be spherical or ovoid intact cystic masses, but often they are irregular and collapsed. The walls vary from extremely thin to a thickness of about 5 mm. The inner surface may be smooth or corrugated. Yellow mural nodules of cholesterol may project into the cavity. The fluid contents are usually brown from the breakdown of blood and when cholesterol crystals are present they impart a shimmering gold or straw colour.

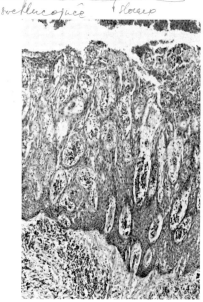

Fig. 73. Proliferating epithelium lining a radicular cyst. HE; ×50.

Almost all radicular cysts are lined wholly or in part by stratified squamous epithelium. These linings may be discontinuous in part and range in thickness from 1 to 50 cell layers. The majority are between 6 and 20 cell layers thick. The epithelial linings may be proliferating and show arcading with an intense associated inflammatory process (*Fig.* 73) or be quiescent and fairly regular with a certain degree of differentiation (*Fig.* 72). Orthokeratinized and parakeratinized linings are very rarely seen in radicular cysts. When they do occur, they are quite different morphologically from those seen in primordial cysts (*see Fig.* 1, p. 5).

103

Secretory characteristics, in the form of mucus cells or ciliated cells, are frequently found in the epithelial linings (Shear, 1960b; Browne, 1972). Mucus cells occurred in as many as 40 per cent of Browne's series of radicular cysts. They may be present in the surface layer of a stratified squamous epithelial lining, either as a continuous row (*Fig. 74*) or as scattered cells; and they may be found associated with ciliated epithelium (*Fig. 75*). They are found in cysts occurring in all parts of the mandible and maxilla. Browne made the interesting observation that there is an increasing incidence of mucus cells with age, the incidence increasing 7 per cent per decade.

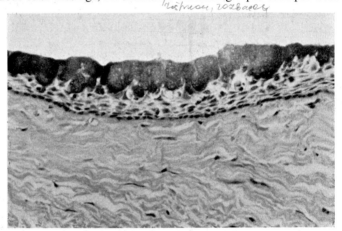

Fig. 74. Mucous cells in the surface layer of the stratified squamous epithelial lining of a radicular cyst. HE; ×225.

Most of the cases in which ciliated epithelium is found occur in the maxilla, but ciliated epithelium has been found in cysts in the anterior and posterior regions of the mandible. The presence of secretory epithelium in radicular cysts, particularly those in the mandible, is probably the result of metaplasia. Some cyst linings with these characteristics show features similar to those described by Fell (1957) in the process of metaplasia from stratified squamous to ciliated epithelium in explants of chick embryo skin grown under the influence of excess vitamin A.

In approximately 10 per cent of radicular cysts, hyaline bodies, often referred to as Rushton's hyaline bodies, are found in the epithelial linings (*Fig. 76*). Only very rarely are they present in the fibrous capsule. The bodies measure up to about 0·1 mm and are linear, straight or curved or of hair-pin shape and sometimes they are concentrically laminated. They are brittle and frequently fracture. Circular or polycyclic bodies are also seen with a clear outer layer surrounding a central granular body.

104

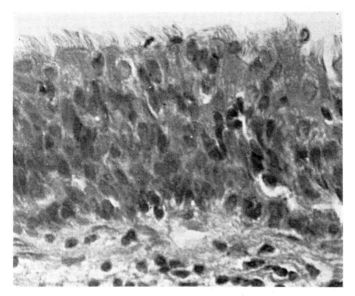

Fig. 75. Ciliated epithelium in a radicular cyst. HE; ×575.

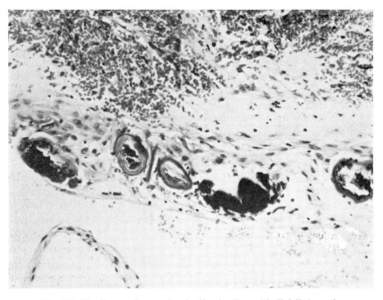

Fig. 76. Hyaline and granular bodies in the epithelial lining of a radicular cyst. HE; ×170.

105

Rushton (1955) believed that the hyaline bodies resemble, in appearance and the liability to fracture, the keratinized secondary enamel cuticle of Gottlieb. My own histochemical studies (Shear, 1961b) indicated that they contained cystine and I suggested that they were of odontogenic epithelial origin and probably a form of keratin. Wertheimer et al. (1962) also found histochemical similarities to keratin but pointed out that the correspondence was not complete. On the other hand, Bouyssou and Guilhem (1965) and Sedano and Gorlin (1968) believed that hyaline bodies are of haematogenous origin; that they are derived from thrombi in venules of the connective tissue which have become varicose and strangled by epithelial cuffs which encircle them; and that they react histochemically as haemoglobin. They suggested that the thrombi shrink centrifugally and undergo splitting, or they may calcify. Dent and Wertheimer (1967) stated however that although hyaline bodies react to several haemoglobin and iron stains, the histochemical reactions for haemoglobin are not specific. I have found that hyaline bodies give a faint reaction with Pickworth's benzidine method for haemoglobin while a control of human erythrocytes stain intensely. Although I agree that the circular or polycyclic forms are sometimes of a morphology which suggests that they are lying in a transversely sectioned blood vessel, there are some puzzling features about their distribution if they are of vascular and haematogenous origin. For one thing they are often seen in epithelium overlying connective tissue devoid of any blood vessels. For another, they are very rarely found in the fibrous capsules, and I have never seen them in this situation. Thirdly, if their pathogenesis is as described, it is most surprising that they do not occur in other situations, but as far as I am aware they have not been described other than in jaw cysts. I have not seen them in nasopalatine duct cysts which are not of odontogenic origin.

Ultrastructural studies of the bodies (Allison, 1974; Jensen and Erickson, 1974; Morgan and Johnson, 1974) have been done on material recovered from paraffin blocks and from reserve tissue stored in formalin. The investigation of Morgan and Johnson failed to demonstrate any close relationships between the bodies and either red cells or blood vessels. They were also unable to demonstrate any cellular structures, or evidence of either cell stratification, desmosomes, or, except in one case, filamentous laminae. In this exceptional instance, they felt that there might be some similarity to the contents of poorly keratinizing epithelial cells. On the whole, however, they believed that their ultrastructural findings ruled out a keratinous origin. They were not able to exclude the possibility that the hyaline bodies represented a type of dental cuticle. Their conclusion was that the bodies are a secretory product of odontogenic epithelium deposited on the surface of particulate matter such as cell debris or cholesterol crystals in a manner analogous to the formation of dental cuticle on the unerupted portions of enamel surfaces. Later enzyme histochemical studies (Morgan and Heyden, 1975) lent support to this theory. Jensen and Erickson ruled out the possibility that the bodies might be composed of keratin or the secondary enamel cuticle. Their observations were unable to support a haematogenous origin.

The presence of hyaline bodies may be suspected if, in examining the gross specimen, the pathologist sees small smooth white dome-shaped swellings of the epithelial surface protruding into the cyst cavity.

Deposits of cholesterol crystals are found in many radicular cysts, but by no means in all (Shear, 1963b; Browne, 1971b; Trott and Esty, 1972). In my own series they were present in 28·5 per cent of cases, and in Trott and Esty's, 30 per cent, whereas Browne reported an incidence of 43·5 per cent in his larger sample. It is likely, however, that if entire cyst linings were examined instead of random sections, the incidence would be higher. Browne has demonstrated a statistically significant correlation ($P < 1$ per cent) between the presence of cholesterol and haemosiderin. He postulated that the main source of cholesterol is that which is released from disintegrating red blood cells in a form which readily crystallizes in the tissues. Cholesterol from this source and also from serum accumulates in the tissues because of the relative inaccessibility of normal lymphatic drainage. Arwill and Heyden (1973) confirmed the origin from red blood cells. They showed that the crystals may form in congested capillaries in the inflamed areas as they appear to be enveloped by endothelial cells.

Trott et al. (1973) supported the finding of a close correlation between the occurrence of cholesterol and haemosiderin-containing macrophages as well as free haemosiderin in the tissues. Their regression analysis showed, however, that only 35 per cent of the cholesterol may be formed from this association. They suggested that slow but considerable accumulation of cholesterol could occur through degeneration and disintegration of lymphocytes, plasma cells and macrophages taking part in the inflammatory process, with consequent release of cholesterol from their walls.

The possibility that circulating plasma lipids are a further source of cholesterol in cysts as they are in atherosclerosis must also be considered. A mechanism similar to that which is thought might occur in atheroma may operate (Shear, 1963b). Beta-lipoproteins in the plasma pass through the fragile thin-walled blood vessels in the inflamed portions of cyst wall in the same manner as the extravasating erythrocytes. There, the beta-lipoproteins split into cholesterol and its esters which are retained, and other lipid components such as phospholipids which are absorbed by the lymphatics.

Once the cholesterol crystals have been deposited in the fibrous capsules of the cysts, they behave as foreign bodies and excite a foreign-body giant-cell reaction. Arwill and Heyden suggested that these giant cells are derived from pericytes of the vessel wall. In histological sections the cholesterol crystals have been dissolved out and clefts are seen surrounded by dense aggregations of multi-nucleate giant cells. The cholesterol masses are extruded from the

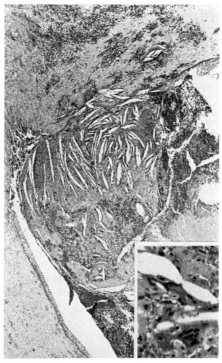

Fig. 77. Mural nodule of cholesterol-containing granulation tissue fungating into the cavity of a radicular cyst. HE; ×24. *Inset:* Multinucleate foreign body giant cells on the surface of the cholesterol clefts. HE; ×150.

fibrous wall by the foreign body reaction. Invariably, the path of least resistance is into the cyst cavity as the external surface of the cyst may consist of dense fibrous tissue, bone and mucosa. When the reaction reaches the epithelial lining, this ulcerates. The granulation tissue containing the cholesterol fungates into the cyst cavity and appears macroscopically and microscopically as a 'mural nodule' (*Fig.*77). Once the entire mass has passed into the cavity the epithelial breach heals and the cholesterol crystals lie free in the cyst fluid (Shear, 1963b).

108

The fibrous capsule of radicular cysts is composed mainly of condensed collagen peripherally and a loose connective tissue adjacent to the epithelial lining. Varying intensities of acute and chronic inflammatory cell infiltrate are present, particularly sub-epithelially. Acute inflammatory cells are seen particularly when the epithelium is proliferating. Usually, however, a chronic inflammatory cell infiltrate features in the fibrous capsule. Russell bodies are seen in about 50 per cent of cases. Remnants of odontogenic epithelium and occasional satellite microcysts may be found. Some cyst walls are markedly vascular. Haemorrhage is invariably present and haemosiderin deposits are seen in many specimens (Shear, 1963c).

Calcifications of various kinds are frequently present. Amorphous calcifications and trabeculae of woven bone occur most commonly and occasionally lamellar bone is found.

Frithiof and Hägglund (1966) examined 12 radicular cysts ultrastructurally. They found wide structural variations between specimens probably ascribable to differences in the degree of inflammation. In their ultrastructural study, Hansen and Kobayasi (1970a) found that the epithelium did not show the regular stratification usually seen in squamous epithelium. They described the presence of 'dark' and 'bright' cells. The dark cells they regarded as undergoing autolysis as they have a dense osmiophilic cytoplasm with indistinguishable organelles and they contain fat droplets, vacuoles and annular structures. Their nucleoplasm is dense and there are clumped chromatin masses. These cells also have poorly developed intercellular connections. The bright cells, on the other hand, have more distinct organelles, numerous mitochondria, ribosomes, granular endoplasmic reticulum and lysosomes, and are probably actively functioning cells.

Carcinomatous Change
A few well-documented cases have been reported which indicate that squamous carcinoma may occasionally arise from the epithelial lining of radicular and other odontogenic cysts. One such case, arising in a residual radicular cyst, was reported by Kay and Kramer (1962) while the case of Ward and Cohen (1963) appears, from their published photomicrograph, to have originated in a primordial cyst. Examples occurring in a radicular and in a dentigerous cyst were illustrated by Pindborg and Hjørting-Hansen (1974). Eversole et al. (1975) reviewed series of cases of central epidermoid carcinoma and central muco-epidermoid carcinoma of the jaws. They found that 75 per cent of the former were associated with a cyst lining and 48 per cent of the latter were associated with either a cyst or an impacted tooth.

Before the diagnosis of carcinoma arising from a cyst lining can be established, a number of alternative possibilities must be excluded (Kay and Kramer, 1962). It is possible that cyst and neoplasm may have developed independently adjacent to one another and ultimately fused in some parts. Careful questioning of the patient and clinical examination are necessary to exclude the possibility that the neoplasm arose primarily from the oral mucosa, or that it is a metastatic deposit in the jaw. A further possibility to be considered is that the lesion was initially an epithelial neoplasm which underwent secondary cystic change.

Despite the undoubted examples which occur from time to time, the incidence of neoplastic change is exceptionally rare in relation to the large numbers of cysts which are seen. Browne and Gough (1972) have suggested that keratin metaplasia in long-standing radicular and dentigerous cysts may precede carcinomatous transformation and examples of epithelial dysplasia are occasionally seen in jaw cysts (see Figs. 14, 15, 16, pp. 20, 21). There is no evidence however that cyst epithelium is at particular risk and there is therefore no justification for regarding cysts as precancerous lesions.

Immunological Studies on Radicular Cysts

Electrophoretic studies of the fluids of radicular and other non-keratinizing cysts have shown that more than half display levels of gamma-globulin much higher than the patients' own serum (Toller and Holborow, 1969; Toller, 1970a). In 19 cyst fluids in which levels of IgG, IgA and IgM were measured independently, all three were significantly raised in most of the non-keratinizing cysts. Immuno-fluorescent staining showed that lymphoid cell aggregates in the walls of radicular cysts often include numerous immunoglobulin-containing cells of the plasma cell series, many of them producing IgG, IgA or IgM, but IgA-staining cells were predominant. These immunoglobulin-producing cells appear to be actively mobile and even capable of penetrating several layers of intact epithelial cells, thereby entering the cyst cavities. Toller believed that this evidence suggests that there is an antigenic stimulus in the cyst wall and in the absence of demonstrable infection either the occult epithelium or its breakdown products are antigenic. This may, he suggested, be the mechanism whereby cysts undergo spontaneous regression. Those people who have a particular tendency to develop cysts may have an ineffective immunological surveillance and suppression mechanism. The question of regression of radicular cysts is discussed further below, in the section on their treatment.

Treatment

Radicular cysts may be treated by marsupialization or by enucleation followed by either open treatment or primary closure. Marsupialization and enucleation procedures have been described in detail by Fickling (1965) and in most standard textbooks of oral surgery. Objections have been raised to treating very large cysts by enucleation and/or primary closure. These are that a large blood clot in the cavity will not organize completely and may become infected; that enucleation may damage adjacent structures or may lead to fractures of the jaw; and that there may be incomplete bone regeneration in the defect with subsequent changes in jaw contour. A careful evaluation by Van Doorn (1972) of a series of 209 jaw cysts treated by enucleation and primary closure showed however that favourable results may be obtained by this procedure irrespective of the size provided that what he terms 'optimal primary closure' is obtained.

Hjørting-Hansen (1970) has detailed the selective indications for implantation of bone in the treatment of cystic jaw lesions. Egyedi and Beyazit (1973) have reported a series of 63 large cysts of the maxilla treated by opening into the nose and/or maxillary antrum. Although the lining was not removed in the majority of cases, follow-up planimetric studies on radiographs of 32 patients showed significant reduction in size in 27.

The non-vital tooth responsible for the cyst should be extracted or root-filled following an apicoectomy.

Oehlers (1970) believed that many periapical lesions left in situ, including cysts, are eliminated by the body once the causative agents are removed. This view was supported by Bhaskar (1972) who suggested that the vast majority of radicular cysts undergo resolution following conservative endodontic therapy. His hypothesis was based on endodontists' claims that 85–90 per cent of apical lesions disappear or become markedly reduced in size following conservative endodontic procedures. As available statistics indicate that 40–50 per cent of all apical lesions are radicular cysts and as it is difficult to distinguish between apical granulomas and radicular cysts on radiographs alone, Bhaskar concluded that the majority of radicular cysts can undergo resolution following root canal therapy and do not require surgical intervention. He suggested that during the endodontic procedure, instrumentation should be done slightly beyond the apical foramen. This produces a transitory acute inflammation which may destroy the epithelial linings of the radicular cysts and convert them into granulomas, thus leading to their resolution. Although clinicians may be tempted by such an hypothesis, I would be reluctant to recommend that the procedure be adopted until further and direct evidence is available that radicular cysts resolve when treated in this way; and at least that it is possible to observe the patients' progress by regular radiographic follow-up.

CHAPTER 12

SIMPLE BONE CYST (TRAUMATIC, HAEMORRHAGIC BONE CYST)

THE simple bone cyst, which occurs in the mandible and practically never in the maxilla, is very similar and probably identical to the solitary or unicameral bone cyst which is most frequently located in the metaphyses at the upper end of the humerus and the femur in children and adolescents.

Clinical Features

Frequency

The simple bone cyst is not a common lesion. We have only 8 specimens in our departmental records although other cases have been treated in the clinical departments of our hospital without any contents having been found for histological examination. In view of the rarity of the lesion, the review published by Howe in 1965 is most valuable, and will be extensively quoted here. His material consisted of 6 of his own cases and 54 from the literature published over the period 1929–63.

The well documented series of 23 cases of Killey and Kay (1972), the 66 cases of Hansen et al. (1974), as well as the reviews of Mayer et al. (1967) and Huebner and Turlington (1971), all provide valuable data on the condition.

In determining which cases to include, Howe used the following criteria. The cyst should be single, have no epithelial lining and show no evidence of acute or prolonged infection. It should contain principally fluid and not soft tissue and the walls should be of bone which is hard though possibly thin in parts.

Age

The solitary bone cyst occurs in young individuals. The age distribution of the 60 patients included in Howe's analysis is shown in *Fig.* 78. The patients ranged in age from $2\frac{1}{2}$ to 35 years and 46 of the 60 (78 per cent) were in their second decade. Killey and Kay also recorded a peak incidence in the second decade, but one patient was over 50 and another over 60. In the series of Hansen et al. the age range was 7 to 75 years and more than half were in the second decade. In our own material, the oldest patient was 40 years of age.

112

Sex

Thirty-six cases in Howe's analysis were recorded in males and 23 in females, a male : female ratio of 1·6 : 1. Killey and Kay, however, reported an incidence of 13 females and 10 males and there was an equal sex distribution in the series of Mayer et al. and Hansen et al. Six of our 8 patients were females.

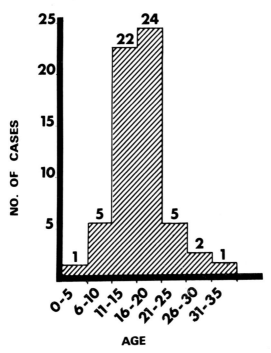

Fig. 78. Age distribution of 60 patients with simple bone cysts of the jaws. (*After Howe, 1965.*)

Site

Simple bone cysts of the jaws occur most frequently in the mandible and Howe stated that only one atypical case had been reported in the maxilla. This was confirmed by Mayer et al. In the more recent report of Hansen et al. (1974) however, about one-third occurred in the maxilla.

Almost all the maxillary cases and the majority of the mandibular cases involved the anterior regions.

Clinical Presentation

In Howe's survey, the majority of cases (60 per cent) were diagnosed fortuitously and almost all of these were chance radiographic findings. Swelling was the presenting symptom in 27 per cent, pain in 10 per cent, while 2 per cent complained of labial paraesthesia and in 2 per cent there were both pain and swelling. Over half the patients gave a history of significant trauma to the area and the time-lag between injury and diagnosis varied from 1 month to 20 years. Howe felt that trauma may play a role in at least some cases.

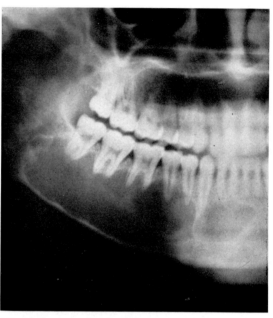

Fig. 79. Radiograph of a simple bone cyst involving an extensive area in the right body of mandible. This example has a well-defined margin with cortication. Interradicular scalloping is a prominent feature. (*Courtesy of Dr. C. J. Nortjé.*)

On clinical examination, 35 per cent had a mandibular swelling, most frequently buccal and labial, and only occasionally lingual. The related teeth were all vital in 67 per cent of cases. Of the 61 patients in the series reported by Hansen et al., 44 were completely symptomless and only 8 reported definite symptoms.

Radiological Features (Fig. 79)

Careful interpretation of good radiographs is most valuable in the diagnosis. The cyst appears as a radiolucent area with an irregular but definite edge and slight cortication. An occlusal view shows the radiolucency extending along cancellous bone.

114

SIMPLE BONE CYST

There is usually little effect on the buccal and lingual plates (Poyton and Morgan, 1965). Of the reviewed cases, 63 per cent showed some degree of marginal condensation but not as sharp or opaque as with radicular cysts. The radiological appearances of lesions in different parts of the mandible are similar. In 72 per cent of cases, usually in the posterior mandible, the cyst enveloped the roots of erupted teeth. Scalloping is a prominent feature of simple bone cysts and occurs both between teeth and away from teeth. The lamina dura may or may not be lost and occasional root resorption may occur. Trabeculation is rare.

Pathogenesis

The pathogenesis of the simple bone cyst is not known but there are a number of theories which have been examined. In 1951, Olech and co-workers suggested the following possible pathogenesis, based upon a traumatic aetiology, and Howe proposed an essentially similar natural history. Olech et al. introduced their hypothesis with the premise that following trauma to a bone, which causes intramedullary haemorrhage, only a failure of early organization of the haematoma in some of the marrow spaces and subsequent liquefaction of the clot can lead to the formation of a traumatic cyst. The crucial point therefore, is the explanation of this failure. The assumptions which these authors postulated appeared to explain, they believed, all the peculiar features of the pathogenesis, location and age incidence of the simple bone cysts. These cysts seem to develop only after injury to those areas of a bone where spongy bone containing haemo-poietic marrow is enclosed in a heavy compact cortical layer. This would explain the most frequent sites in the metaphyses of long bones and in the mandible. It would also explain the fact that most simple bone cysts develop in young individuals.

Although there are arguments against the proposal, it seems that at least in some cases trauma may be the initiating factor. Trauma, or some other stimulus, leads to rupture of thin-walled sinusoids and intramedullary haemorrhage occurs.

According to Olech et al., the primary haematoma will not be organized if it is not in contact with reactive and fibrous connective tissue and this will not be present if the intramedullary haemorrhage has led to necrosis of the bone marrow itself and related endosteum. The trabeculae of medullary bone are then slowly resorbed by osteoclastic activity on their opposite surfaces and by the time the viable connective tissue gains contact with the haematoma, the latter has liquefied. The breakdown of haematomas and their failure to organize, particularly if they are large, is however a well-known problem in surgery and it is perfectly conceivable that this

115

can occur following intramedullary haemorrhage even in the presence of reactive and fibrous connective tissue.

Although the majority of simple bone cysts are found at operation to contain only air or some other gas, the fact that some contain blood or serosanguineous fluid tends to support the concept of a haematoma breaking down. The breakdown products of haemolysis produce a local rise in osmotic pressure. Toller (1964) has confirmed experimentally that the osmotic tension of a simple bone cyst fluid was greater than that of the patient's blood. This in turn leads to a transudation into the cyst fluid. In the presence of intact cortical bone there is an increase in intraosseous pressure which leads to resorption of bone by osteoclastic activity and sometimes swelling by concurrent periosteal bone deposition. Occasional tooth displacement occurs. As transudation into the cysts occurs, the fluid is diluted so that intracystic pressure drops, but further bleeds may be responsible for progression of the lesion. Once no more bleeding occurs there will be gradual absorption of the serous fluid in the cavity, which becomes empty. The fact that they are practically never found in patients over 30 years suggests that they are self-limiting and undergo spontaneous regression. When the space is filled with blood as a result of surgical intervention, the defect heals and it has been suggested that a spontaneous haemorrhage into an empty cyst cavity may do the same.

This, however, is the main problem in accepting the pathogenesis described above. Essentially it proposes that on the one hand, intrabony haemorrhage is responsible for initiating and then maintaining the process, whereas on the other hand haemorrhage into the cyst cavity in the course of treatment leads to ready repair, and spontaneous haemorrhage is postulated as the reason for resolution without treatment. Olech et al. explained this by the fact that the new blood clot which fills the cyst cavity is in contact with healthy connective tissue of the flap from which the organization of the clot commences. When a pathological fracture occurs through a simple bone cyst, they suggested that the reason for the cyst healing is not only the formation of a fresh blood clot, but also its contact with the vital connective tissue of the periosteum. Although no further evidence as to the pathogenesis of the simple bone cyst has been published in the years since the paper by Olech and his colleagues, there are nevertheless aspects of their hypothesis which require further elucidation and I should like to see some experimental evidence that similar cysts can be produced by trauma.

Pathology

When the cyst cavities are opened at operation, they are frequently found to be empty. In the other cases, blood, serosanguineous or serous fluid may be present. In 58 per cent of Howe's sample, no visible lining was seen and in the other cases either a thin membrane, granulation tissue or blood clot were described.

Histological Features

The simple bone cyst consists of a loose vascular fibrous tissue membrane of variable thickness with no epithelial lining, although fragments of fibrin with enmeshed red cells may be seen. Haemorrhage and haemosiderin pigment are usually present and scattered small multinucleate cells are often found (*Fig.* 80). Some cyst walls, possibly cases of longer standing, are more densely fibrous. The adjacent bone, when included in the specimen, shows osteoclastic resorption on its inner surface.

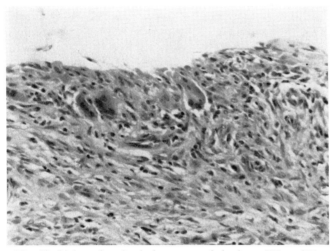

Fig. 80. Lining of a simple bone cyst of the jaw. HE; ×215.

Treatment

Surgical treatment is usually recommended because when the cavity is opened, and haemorrhage encouraged, rapid obliteration of the lesion results. If, however, the simple bone cyst does heal spontaneously, the need for surgical intervention may well be questioned provided that an accurate diagnosis can be established on clinical and radiological grounds and that the patient is able to attend for follow-up radiographs at yearly intervals. Four patients in the series of Killey and Kay refused surgical treatment and follow-up radiographs over a period of years have shown spontaneous regeneration of bone and eventual disappearance of the radiolucent areas in all cases. These authors felt, however, that spontaneous regression in cases of the expansile variety is unlikely.

117

DEVELOPMENTAL LINGUAL SALIVARY GLAND DEPRESSION OF THE MANDIBLE

(Stafne cavity/Static bone cavity/Latent bone cyst)

The developmental lingual salivary gland depression of the mandible (*Fig.* 81) is not a cyst. It does however produce a cystic appearance on radiographs, and as it is occasionally confused with the simple bone cyst a brief note on the entity is included here. Of importance in the differential diagnosis is that the simple bone cyst almost invariably lies above the inferior alveolar canal while the salivary gland depression lies below the canal.

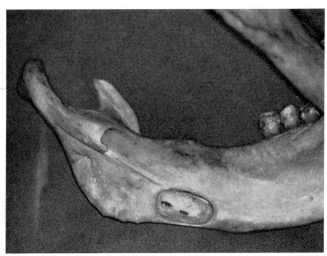

Fig. 81. Developmental lingual salivary gland depression of the mandible. (*Courtesy of Professor P. V. Tobias.*)

A description of 35 cases was reported by Stafne in 1942 and since then the features have become well documented. The cavities are usually discovered fortuitously during radiographic examination. They appear as round or ovoid radiolucencies varying from 1 to 3 cm diameter below the inferior alveolar canal approximately in line with the position of the third molar tooth (*Fig.* 82). Fordyce (1956) pointed out that apart from the outer distinct cortication, a second inner ring could frequently also be identified which encircles an area of more marked radiolucency.

Surgical exploration of these cavities has indicated that they represent developmental defects on the lingual aspects of the mandible which are occupied by a lobe of normal submandibular

118

salivary gland. The defects are not necessarily congenital. Tolman and Stafne (1967) have shown that radiological evidence of their development may first appear after the patients have reached

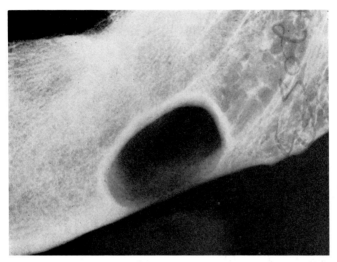

Fig. 82. Radiograph of dry mandible illustrated in *Fig.* 81. (*Courtesy of Dr. H. Mirels.*)

middle age. Although they may develop slowly and progressively, there is no indication at the present time that they ever reach a size large enough to warrant surgical intervention.

119

CHAPTER 13

ANEURYSMAL BONE CYST

THE aneurysmal bone cyst is an uncommon lesion which has been found in most bones of the skeleton, although the majority occur in the long bones and in the spine (Clough and Price, 1968). The term 'aneurysmal bone cyst' was suggested by Jaffe and Lichtenstein (1942) to describe the characteristic 'blow out' of the bone seen in radiographs of the lesion.

Clinical Features

Frequency

Aneurysmal bone cyst of the jaws is extremely rare and we have only one case in our records. The first report of these cysts involving the craniofacial skeleton appears to be that of Bernier and Bhaskar (1958). In the following year, Bhaskar et al. described 5 cases. Gruskin and Dahlin reviewed the literature in 1968, and reported 13 cases including two of their own. A few cases have been reported since (Byrd et al., 1969; Daugherty and Eversole, 1971; Oliver, 1973). Daugherty and Eversole reviewed 17 cases including their own and the data for age, sex and site recorded below, are derived from their paper.

Age

Except for one case in a female of 59, all were in the age range 6–22. Most cases occurred in children and adolescents, an age distribution similar to that for aneurysmal cysts in other bones.

Sex

Six cases occurred in males and 10 in females. The sex of one patient had not been recorded.

Site

Eleven of the 17 cases were in the mandible. Most of these were in the posterior part of the body or involved the angle or ascending ramus. One of the cases reported by Bhaskar et al. (1959) occurred in the maxillary canine-premolar region and resembled a globulo-maxillary cyst.

Clinical Presentation
Aneurysmal cysts of the jaws produce firm, usually painless swellings although pain is a feature of the cysts in other bones, often following a pathological fracture. In some of the recorded cases, the swelling and malocclusion became progressively worse. Occasionally there is a history of recent migration of teeth. Bruits are not heard.

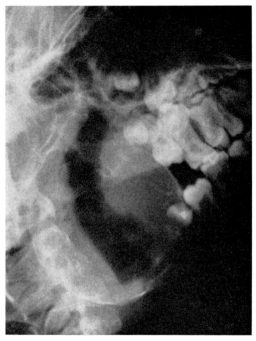

Fig. 83. Radiograph of an aneurysmal bone cyst in the angle and ascending ramus of the mandible. There is a ballooning expansion of the cortex. (*Courtesy of Dr. I. Rosenberg.*)

Radiological Features
The aneurysmal bone cyst produces a radiolucent area which expands the bone and may balloon the cortex and which is usually unilocular (*Fig.* 83). Others, however, are described as having faintly discernible septation, or trabeculations, and some are described as multilocular or honeycomb-like.

Pathogenesis
The pathogenesis is not known although there are a number of theories. Although trauma has been postulated, there is little evidence to support it. The most favoured view is that the cyst

121

results from a vascular disturbance in the form of sudden venous occlusion or the development of an arteriovenous shunt. This would usually occur in more vascular, newly-formed parts of the immature skeleton and possibly arising, in some cases at least, in a pre-existing lesion (Clough and Price, 1968). These latter authors described two cases, one of which contained areas with the appearance of fibrous dysplasia and the other with features of chondromyxoid fibroma. Our own case had solid areas which were histologically indistinguishable from ossifying fibroma and parts of this are obviously undergoing cystic degeneration (*Figs.* 84 and 85). I have seen a similar

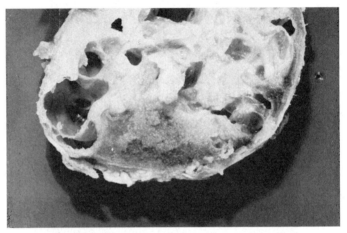

Fig. 84. Section through part of a gross specimen of an aneurysmal bone cyst of the mandible. Solid areas are interspersed with multiple cysts or locules.

picture in two cases circulated by the WHO International Reference Centre for the Histological Definition and Classification of Odontogenic Tumours, Jaw Cysts and Allied Lesions, and the case reported by Oliver (1973) appears to be similar. Two other of the WHO cases are very suggestive of origin in a central giant cell granuloma of the jaws (*Fig.* 86), because there are extensive areas of solid tumour in parts of the lesion. These findings lead me to believe that there is support for the concept that at least some cases of aneurysmal bone cyst develop in pre-existing lesions.

Pathology

At operation an intact periosteum and a very thin shell of bone usually covers the cyst. When this is removed, dark venous blood wells up. Bleeding may be profuse and difficult to control until the cyst has been removed. The cyst contains variable amounts of soft tissue consisting of friable vascular tissue which subdivides the cavity into a number of blood-filled locules (*Fig.* 84). Part of the lesion may contain areas of more solid tissue. These may represent either areas of repair or remnants of a pre-existing lesion. No direct communication with any vessels can be demonstrated at operation.

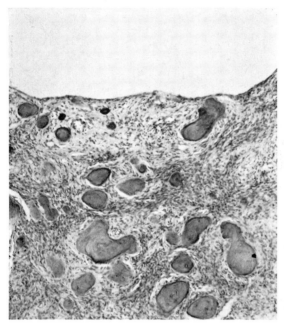

Fig. 85. Aneurysmal bone cyst of the mandible. The solid areas show the features of ossifying fibroma and portion of one of the many locules is present at the top of the photomicrograph. HE; ×75.

Histological Features

The lesions consist of many capillaries and blood-filled spaces of varying size lined by flat spindle cells and separated by delicate loose-textured fibrous tissue containing small multinucleate cells and scattered trabeculae of osteoid and woven bone. In some of the solid areas, sheets of vascular tissue, containing large numbers of multinucleate giant cells, fibroblasts, haemorrhage and haemosiderin, look very much like giant cell granuloma of the jaws (*Fig.* 86). Other solid areas may have the appearance of fibrous dysplasia, ossifying fibroma (*Fig.* 85) and possibly other jaw tumours, and this gives credence to the view that the aneurysmal bone cyst may represent secondary change in a pre-existing lesion. The blood-filled spaces have no elastic tissue or smooth muscle around them,

123

which indicates that they do not represent dilated blood vessels. Mitoses may be quite numerous but are of normal pattern and are seen among groups of cells rather than dispersed through the tissue. There are no cellular features suggestive of malignant neoplasia (Clough and Price, 1968).

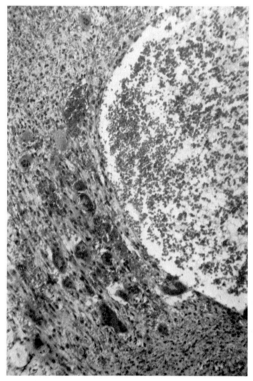

Fig. 86. Aneurysmal bone cyst in which the solid areas have histological features identical to those of the central giant cell granuloma of the jaws. HE; ×80.

Treatment

The aneurysmal bone cyst is a benign condition but may recur after incomplete curettage. Even after careful curettage and bone grafting, Clough and Price (1968) reported continued growth in 4 of 6 cases. They recommended complete excision provided that this would not interfere with function. Failing this, thorough curettage and bone grafting, repeated if necessary, should be done. There is no place for radiotherapy in the treatment of jaw lesions.

CHAPTER 14

CYSTS ASSOCIATED WITH THE MAXILLARY ANTRUM

THERE are two cysts which are considered under this heading: the benign mucosal cyst of the maxillary antrum which occurs fairly frequently, and the surgical ciliated cyst of the maxilla which appears to be very rare.

BENIGN MUCOSAL CYST OF THE MAXILLARY ANTRUM

The mucosal cyst of the maxillary antrum has also been referred to as a mucocele or retention cyst and uncertainty as to its pathogenesis has led in the past to its being termed 'mesothelial' cyst and 'lymphangiectatic' cyst.

Clinical Features

Frequency

This cyst probably occurs more commonly than was previously thought. Kwapis and Whitten (1971) have pointed out that more of them are being revealed with the increased use of panoramic radiographs of the maxilla. Their survey of a series of such radiographs disclosed the presence of round radio-opaque areas in the maxillary sinuses of 22 patients. Surgical exploration and subsequent histological examination were carried out on 14 of these and the features were consistent with the diagnosis of mucosal cyst of the maxillary sinus. Myall et al. (1974) surveyed 1469 orthopantographs and made a radiological diagnosis of mucosal antral cyst in 75 cases (5·1 per cent).

Age

In the survey of Myall et al. referred to above, 19 of the 75 patients were younger than 21. The peak incidence, consisting of 33 cases, occurred in the age group 21–30 years. In the subsequent three decades, 11, 6 and 4 patients were found, respectively, and 2 patients were over 60 years (*Fig.* 87).

Sex

Fifty of the 75 cysts reported by Myall et al. occurred in males.

Site

In the series of Myall et al., 43 of the 75 cases involved the antral floor (57 per cent). The cysts developed on the lateral wall in 24 cases (32 per cent) and the other antral surfaces were occasionally involved. In the great majority of cases only single cysts occurred, but in a few instances they were multiple and sometimes bilateral.

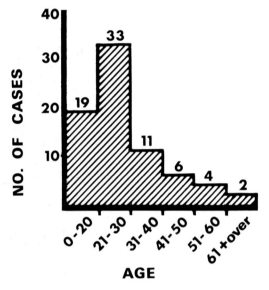

Fig. 87. Age distribution of 75 patients with mucosal cysts of the maxillary antrum. (*After Myall et al., 1974.*)

Clinical Presentation

The mucosal cyst of the maxillary antrum is characterized by the absence of symptoms in most cases and the lesions are usually only discovered in the course of routine radiological examination. Patients occasionally complain of slight discomfort such as a localized dull pain in the antral region, or fullness or numbness of the cheek, nasal obstruction and a copious postnasal discharge if the cyst ruptures (Killey and Kay, 1973). Very occasionally an antral cyst may produce a swelling. One such case from our files occurred in a 32-year-old woman. She had a painless fluctuant swelling of the left maxilla extending from the canine to the second molar which was noticed by her dentist during routine dental examination. She had not previously had any surgical procedure in the region. At operation a cyst was found arising from the lateral wall of the maxillary antrum and a diagnosis of retention cyst of the antrum was made histologically (*see Fig.* 89, p. 128).

126

Radiological Features

The lesions are usually only discovered in the course of routine periapical radiography which includes the involved region. The cysts appear as spherical, ovoid or dome-shaped radio-opacities which have a smooth and uniform outline (*Fig.* 88). They may have a narrow or broad base. They vary in size from minute to very large and may occasionally occupy the entire maxillary sinus (Killey and Kay, 1973). The smooth curved borders are well-defined but not corticated. There is no resorption of adjacent bone and of particular

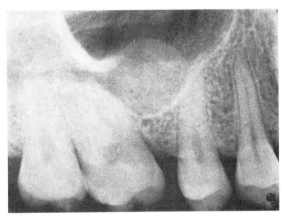

Fig. 88. Radiograph of a mucosal cyst of the maxillary antrum. (*Courtesy of Dr. C. J. Nortjé.*)

importance is the persistence of the thin radio-opaque line of the antral cortex itself (Myall et al.). When an antral cyst is suspected on intraoral radiography, supplementary panoramic radiographs are extremely useful in providing a view of the maxillary sinuses with little superimposition of adjacent structures.

Inflammatory lesions of the sinus must be considered in the differential diagnosis as well as the apical radicular cyst and surgical ciliated cyst of the maxilla.

Follow-up radiological examination has shown that the cyst may persist without a change in size for a long time, and may eventually disappear spontaneously. Others slowly increase in size.

Pathogenesis

The pathogenesis of the mucosal cyst of the antrum has not been definitely determined but a previous infection is frequently implicated. Kwapis and Whitten (1971) have suggested that severe inflammation around the ducts of the mucous glands of the antral lining may alter their integrity. When the patient sneezes, mucus can

127

be expelled into the soft tissues through the wall of such an injured duct. Once this pathway for the extraglandular accumulation of mucus has been established, the process may continue until a cyst has developed.

Pathological Features

When explored surgically, it is possible to demonstrate the intact and undisturbed cyst. It has a smooth blue surface, is thin-walled and contains mucinous material.

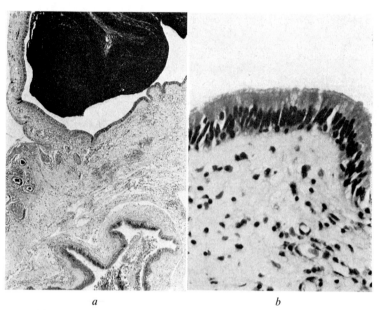

a   *b*

Fig. 89. *a*, Mucosal cyst of the maxillary antrum. The cyst (top) illustrated here is of the secretory variety. It is lined by pseudo-stratified ciliated columnar epithelium and is filled with mucin. The lining of the maxillary antrum is seen below. PAS; ×20. *b*, Mucosal cyst of the maxillary antrum. Higher magnification of part of the cyst lining illustrated in *Fig. 89a*. HE; ×250.

The microscopic features are very much like those of an oral mucocele. Usually no epithelial lining is present but in the case referred to above and illustrated in *Figs. 89a, b*, there was a mucin-containing cyst lined by pseudostratified ciliated columnar epithelium. The connective tissue wall of the cyst is infiltrated with varying numbers of chronic inflammatory cells and the lumen may contain inflammatory cells. The type which are not lined by epithelium are sometimes referred to as non-secretory cysts and those lined by respiratory epithelium as the secretory type of antral cysts (Shafer et al., 1974).

128

Treatment

In view of the fact that most of these cysts remain static and some regress spontaneously, and that they usually cause little discomfort, Kwapis and Whitten (1971) have recommended that surgical intervention is unnecessary. Killey and Kay (1973) tended to agree with this but suggested that if symptoms are present cannulation and drainage may be done. Large cysts, they felt, should be removed through a Caldwell–Luc approach.

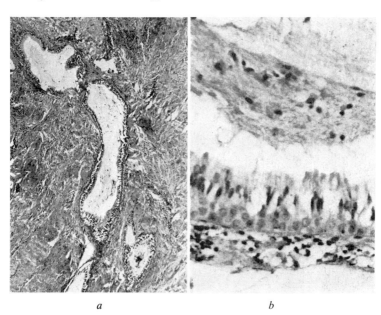

a   *b*

Fig. 90. *a*, Surgical ciliated cyst of the maxilla. The cyst lining which is composed of pseudostratified ciliated columnar epithelium has ramified irregularly. HE; ×32. *b*, Surgical ciliated cyst of the maxilla. Higher magnification of part of lining illustrated in *Fig.* 90*a*. HE; ×270.

SURGICAL CILIATED CYST OF THE MAXILLA

Gregory and Shafer (1958) have drawn attention to the development of cysts in the maxilla in patients whose maxillary sinuses have been opened surgically during a Caldwell–Luc operation. The patients usually complain of poorly localized pain or discomfort in the maxilla. Radiographs reveal a well-defined radiolucent area closely related to the maxillary sinus. Occasionally the cystic area appears to encroach on the sinus itself but lack of communication between the two has been demonstrated by injecting the sinus with a radio-opaque material.

Histologically the cysts are lined by pseudostratified ciliated columnar epithelium, with squamous metaplasia in infected areas (*Figs.* 90*a*, *b*). Gregory and Shafer suggested that the cysts are derived from the epithelial lining of the maxillary sinus which is trapped in the wound during closure of the Caldwell–Luc incision, and subsequently begins to proliferate.

These cysts do not seem to be common, possibly because they are not diagnosed. I have seen one case for which I made this diagnosis in a man aged 49 who had had a Caldwell–Luc operation 11 years before for removal of a tooth from the left maxillary antrum. Radiographs showed a radiolucent expansion of the left maxilla with a radio-opaque margin. A history of a previous Caldwell–Luc procedure is valuable in distinguishing the lesion from a mucous cyst of the maxillary sinus.

CHAPTER 15

DEVELOPMENTAL CYSTS OF THE SOFT TISSUES OF THE MOUTH, FACE AND NECK

DERMOID AND EPIDERMOID CYSTS

DERMOID and epidermoid cysts may occur on the floor of the mouth. Dermoid cysts are lined by epidermis and skin appendages are present in the fibrous wall. Epidermoid cysts are lined by epidermis, but contain no appendages.

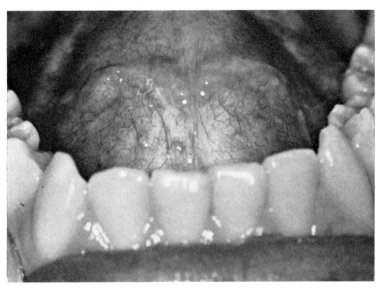

Fig. 91. Dermoid cyst of floor of mouth.

Valuable reviews of these cysts have been written by Meyer (1955) and Seward (1965). They quoted statistics from the Mayo Clinic which indicated that of 1495 dermoid cysts seen over a 25-year period, 24 (1·6 per cent) occurred in the floor of the mouth. Although they may be present at birth and in old patients, the majority occur between the ages of 15 and 35 years. They are equally distributed in males and females.

Most dermoid cysts of the floor of the mouth occur in the midline and are referred to as the median dermoids. They produce swellings of the floor of mouth (*Fig.* 91) and neck. Lateral dermoids are very

131

rare. The intraoral swelling lifts the tongue and may lead to difficulty in speaking, eating or breathing. The swelling in the neck gives the patient a 'double-chin' appearance. The swelling may feel doughy or fluctuant. The lateral dermoid usually produces less swelling than the median. The cysts tend to be small in infancy and enlarge during adolescence. Seward believed that dermoid cysts always originate above the mylohoid muscle, but may penetrate it. They tend to lie close beneath the mucosa of the floor of the mouth. The lateral dermoid develops deep down in the muscular gutter formed by the genioglossus and the hyoglossus medially and the mylohyoid laterally.

The origin of dermoids of the floor of the mouth, like other developmental cysts, is controversial. Having examined and discarded a number of concepts, Seward (1965) suggested, not very confidently, that the most likely site for their origin is anteriorly between the contributions from the mandibular arches to the tongue. Regarding the lateral dermoids, he believed that their anatomical situation indicates an origin from either the ventral end of the first pharyngeal pouch or from the extreme ventral end of the first branchial cleft. The problem with postulating an origin from contributions of mandibular arches to the tongue or from the first pharyngeal pouch is that it implies endodermal derivation. This seems unlikely for a structure which contains skin adnexae. On the other hand, Hamilton and Mossman (1972) stated that by the 30th–32nd day of intra-uterine life, the endoderm of the floor of the mouth can no longer be distinguished from stomodeal ectoderm and there is probably a considerable amount of intermingling of the two epithelia. The boundary line is however behind that part of the epithelium of the mandibular process which gives origin to the teeth.

As already indicated, both dermoid and epidermoid cysts are lined by keratinized epidermis. Occasional cases may have areas of pseudo-stratified ciliated columnar epithelium. The dermoid cysts are characterized by the presence in the wall of one or more dermal appendages such as hair follicles, sweat glands or sebaceous glands (*Fig.* 92). Hair is very rarely found. The lumen is usually filled with keratin.

Treatment is by surgical excision. Seward pointed out that even extensive cysts can be removed through the mouth. If they are very large, partial evacuation of the contents makes removal easier. He suggested however that where a cyst has been inflamed and is likely to be adherent, or where large blood vessels pass near the cyst wall, it may be wise to approach through the neck to avoid complications.

Issa and Davies (1971) have recorded an exceptionally rare example of a dermoid cyst which occurred in the coronoid region of the mandible in a 26-year-old woman.

Implantation keratinizing epidermoid cysts may occur in other parts of the mouth as a result of trauma (Ettinger and Manderson, 1973). These cysts are of limited size and remain small over many years. They are lined by a thin even layer of keratinizing stratified squamous epithelium surrounded by loose collagenous connective tissue. The cyst cavity is filled with keratin.

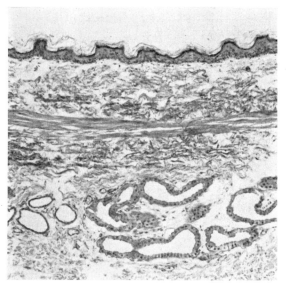

Fig. 92. Dermoid cyst with dermal appendages in the wall. HE; ×75.

Sewerin and Praetorius (1974) described the occurrence of keratin-filled epidermoid cysts of the vermilion border of the lower lip which they believed represent dilated excretory ducts of the sebaceous glands. Serial sectioning of material from their cases revealed an orifice which formed a direct connexion between the cystic cavity and the surface. Consecutive sections also showed a sebaceous gland in the wall at one level and not at another and they emphasized that serial sectioning is obviously necessary before one attempts to label a cyst as either dermoid or epidermoid.

Keratinous cysts may occur on the skin of the face, neck and scalp. Two varieties can be distinguished histologically. The commonest type is the epidermal cyst. These are often produced by traumatic implantation and hence are most frequently found on the hands and fingers. They are lined by keratinized stratified squamous epithelium with a prominent stratum granulosum (*Fig.* 93). When

133

part of the cyst lining ulcerates, a chronic inflammatory cell infiltration and foreign body type multinucleate giant cells are seen in the cyst wall.

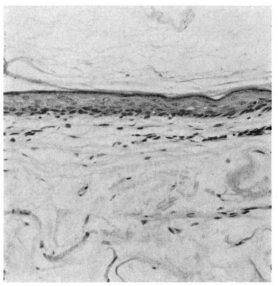

Fig. 93. Epidermal cyst of skin. HE; ×185.

The less common variety of keratinous cyst is the pilar type. These usually occur on the scalp, but rarely may be seen on the face, neck, trunk and extremities. They are lined by a stratified squamous epithelium but no stratum granulosum is formed (*Figs*. 94*a, b*). The superficial epithelial cells are swollen and the keratinization which occurs has been likened to that which is found in the cortex of hair and the proximal third of the follicle without the presence of a granular layer (Ackerman, 1968). The term 'sebaceous cyst' which was used for this lesion is outmoded.

Dermoid cysts sometimes occur on the face. These are called sequestration dermoids. The commonest situation is just above the outer canthus of the eye where it is referred to as the external angular dermoid.

BRANCHIAL CLEFT (LYMPHO-EPITHELIAL) CYST

The commonest location of branchial cleft cysts is superficially in the neck, close to the angle of the mandible, anterior to the sternocleidomastoid muscle. They occur at all ages with a fairly equal distribution from the first to the sixth decades (Rickles and Little, 1967). There is no sex predilection.

134

The neck lesions vary in size from small to very large (about 10 cm diameter). In view of their thick wall and fluid contents they impart, on palpation, a sensation similar to that of a partly-filled hot water bottle.

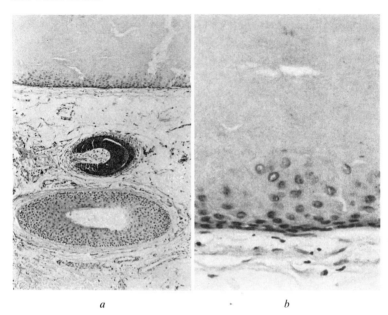

a   *b*

Fig. 94. *a*, Pilar cyst of skin. HE; ×50. *b*, Pilar cyst of skin, showing the swelling of the superficial epithelial cells. HE; ×270.

Less commonly, branchial cleft cysts are found in the floor of the mouth and the tongue. Bhaskar (1966) reported a series of 24 intraoral branchial cysts, 15 of which were in the floor of mouth and 9 in the tongue. Most of the tongue cases involved the lateral margin. The age range was 15–65 years. No case occurred in the first decade and the majority were found in the third, fourth and fifth decades. Males (17 cases) were involved more frequently than females (7 cases). The lesions usually appeared as non-ulcerated, freely movable masses which had been present for periods ranging from 1 month to many years. Schiødt and Friis-Hasché (1972) reviewed the literature and their findings were essentially the same as Bhaskar's. Giunta and Cataldo (1973) reported a series of 21 of their own intraoral cases. The ages of their patients ranged from 7 to 65 years. There were 12 females and 9 males. Seventeen of the cases (80 per cent) involved the floor of the mouth, 2 were in the soft palate and one each in the retromolar area and the mandibular labial vestibule. They ranged in size from 3 to 15 mm in greatest diameter, with an

135

average of 6 mm. More than half of the cases were diagnosed clinically as mucoceles. All were treated by surgical removal without recurrence.

Most workers subscribe to the view that the branchial cyst develops from epithelial remnants of the branchial clefts and pouches. Bhaskar and Bernier (1959) postulated however that the neck cyst is not of 'branchial' origin but that about 96 per cent of

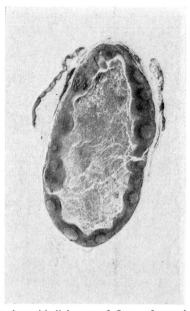

Fig. 95. Lympho-epithelial cyst of floor of mouth. HE; ×6.

them in reality represent cysts in cervical lymph nodes. The cystic change occurs in salivary gland epithelium which is trapped in the nodes of the neck during embryogenesis. They proposed therefore that the lesion should be called 'lympho-epithelial cyst' rather than 'branchial cyst'. Bhaskar (1966) believed that as the oral cavity contains foci of lymphoid tissue it is possible that ectopic glandular epithelium within these foci can undergo similar cystic change and form the lympho-epithelial cyst of the oral cavity. Support for this view comes from Vickers and von der Muhll (1966) who performed surgical autogenous transplants of hamsters' cheek pouch epithelium into their submandibular lymph nodes. In 7 of 9 experimental animals, inclusion cysts lined by keratinized stratified squamous epithelium formed within the lymph nodes.

In a very careful study, Rickles and Little (1967) concluded that several structures may give rise to the epithelium lining these cysts.

The few cysts found in the upper-neck region could develop from either salivary gland inclusions in parotid lymph nodes or from epithelial remnants of the upper portion of the branchial apparatus. The majority of cysts found in the midneck region could develop from epithelial remnants of the cervical sinus and/or the branchial

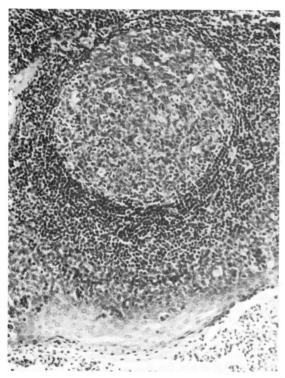

Fig. 96. Higher magnification of lympho-epithelial cyst illustrated in *Fig. 95*. The cyst is lined by stratified squamous epithelium. HE; × 150.

pharyngeal pouches, both of which are part of the branchial apparatus. The cysts found in the lower-neck region may develop from remnants of the thymic duct or from the lower portions of the branchial apparatus.

The branchial cyst in the mouth is lined by stratified squamous epithelium devoid of rete ridges and which may be keratinized. The majority of cysts in the neck are lined by stratified squamous epithelium. Many fewer are lined by ciliated or non-ciliated pseudo-stratified columnar epithelium and a few have a lining of simple cuboidal or flat epithelium (Rickles and Little, 1967). Areas of

137

ulceration occur. The epithelium is closely enveloped by lymphoid tissue in which follicles with germinal centres are characteristically present (*Figs*. 95 and 96).

THYROGLOSSAL DUCT CYST

The anlage of the median lobe of the thyroid gland develops at about the fourth week of intra-uterine life from a site at the base of the tongue which is recognized later as the foramen caecum. A hollow epithelial stalk, known as the thyroglossal duct, extends caudally and passes ventral to the hyoid bone to the ventral aspect of the thyroid cartilage where it joins the developing lateral lobes. The thyroglossal duct disintegrates by about the tenth week, but cysts may form from residues of the duct at any point along its line of descent. There is a high incidence during the first two decades.

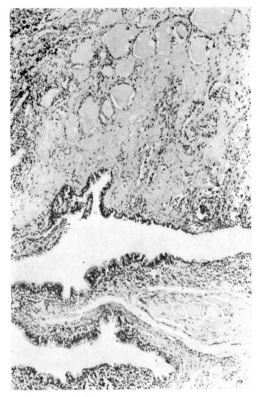

Fig. 97. Thyroglossal duct cyst lined by pseudostratified columnar epithelium. Thyroid tissue is present in the wall. HE; ×70.

The cysts are most commonly located in the area of the hyoid bone, and when they occur in the mouth, they do so either in the floor or at the foramen caecum. A proportion of thyroglossal duct cysts have an associated fistula.

The cysts are usually in the midline and produce soft, movable, sometimes tender swellings. Classically, they lift when the patient swallows or protrudes the tongue.

Histologically, they are lined by a pseudostratified columnar epithelium which may be ciliated, or by a stratified squamous epithelium. The latter type of epithelium is seen particularly in cysts close to the mouth. Thyroid tissue may be seen in the fibrous wall (*Fig.* 97).

ANTERIOR MEDIAN LINGUAL CYST

The anterior medial lingual cyst is a rare lesion. A case was reported by Fink (1963) which occurred in a 5-year-old boy. There was a fluctuant swelling of the anterior half of the dorsum of the tongue. It had been present since birth and had recurred after it had been incised and drained two years before. The cyst was enucleated.

On histological examination, it was lined in different parts by pseudostratified ciliated columnar epithelium and by cuboidal epithelium. The fibrous capsule showed a moderate infiltration of chronic inflammatory cells. A similar case was described by Quinn (1960) in a 9-year-old boy and this was lined by a parakeratinized stratified squamous epithelium.

It was suggested that this cyst develops from epithelium entrapped between the lateral tubercles of the developing tongue. Such cysts may also possibly arise as a result of implantation of epithelium as occurs in epidermoid cysts of the skin.

ORAL CYSTS WITH GASTRIC OR INTESTINAL EPITHELIUM

The rare occurrence of cysts in the mouth containing gastric or intestinal epithelium has been reported from time to time, and Gorlin and Jirasek (1970) have reviewed the literature. Fourteen cases, including one of their own, have been included in their analysis.

Most cases have occurred in infants and young children and two examples in older patients had been present since their childhood. All but two cases occurred in males. The cysts were located in the anterior portion of the tongue in 7 cases, in the posterior portion in 2, in the floor of the mouth in 3, and in the neck in 2.

The cysts may be enclosed entirely within the tongue or floor of mouth or may communicate with the surface.

The origin of the heterotopic gastric and intestinal mucosa is not known. Gorlin and Jirasek pointed out that in the 3–4 mm embryo the undifferentiated primitive stomach lies in the midneck region not far from the anlage of the tongue. Gastric mucosa has been shown to occur in the oesophagus of 7·8 per cent of infants and in 51 per cent of these the heterotopic tissue was located in the upper third. They suggested that in the oral cavity in the sublingual region, and in the region of the apex and dorsum of the tongue, the ectodermal and endodermal epithelia fuse and mix. This may explain the presence of heterotopic gastric or intestinal mucosa.

Microscopically, the cysts may be lined partly by stratified squamous epithelium and partly by gastric mucosa of the type seen in the body and fundus of the stomach. Both parietal and chief cells may be found. Gastric glands may be present. Some cysts have a muscularis mucosa. The cyst reported by Gorlin and Jirasek was lined with intestinal mucosa and Paneth cells, goblet cells and argentaffin cells were demonstrable. Another interesting feature of their case, which occurred on the floor of the mouth, was the presence of a tube which extended from the floor of the mouth into the cyst. The tube was lined by stratified squamous epithelium and adjacent sebaceous glands emptied into the tube.

CHAPTER 16

CYSTS OF THE SALIVARY GLANDS: MUCOUS EXTRAVASATION CYST; MUCOUS RETENTION CYST; RANULA

MUCOUS extravasation cysts and mucous retention cysts are often referred to collectively as mucoceles. Our practice has been to use the term 'mucous extravasation cyst' for those lesions in which mucus has extravasated into the connective tissues and in which there is no epithelial lining. The term 'mucous retention cyst' is employed to describe mucoceles which are lined by epithelium.

Clinical Features

Frequency

Mucoceles of the mouth are very common. Their true incidence is difficult to determine as many patients endure them without seeking treatment, and of those diagnosed a large number are not surgically excised and do not reach a pathology department. Series of cases of mucoceles of the mouth have been reported by Bhaskar et al. (1956b), Standish and Shafer (1959), Gardner et al. (1963), Robinson and Hjørting-Hansen (1964), Cohen (1965), Southam (1974) and Harrison (1975). Our own material consists of 107 cysts in 106 patients during the period 1958–73. Of these, 91 (85 per cent) were extravasation and 16 (15 per cent) were retention cysts. This represents a higher proportion of retention cysts than in the series reported by Standish and Shafer (6·2 per cent of 97), Cohen (9 per cent of 80) and Southam (5·1 per cent of 236 mucoceles), but similar to that of Chaudhry et al. (1960) (16·5 per cent of 66) and Robinson and Hjørting-Hansen (17·6 per cent of 125).

Age

The ages of the patients at diagnosis in a series of 80 of our cases is shown in *Fig. 98*. The youngest patient was 7 and the oldest 88 years, with a peak incidence in the third decade. Other studies have shown a peak incidence in the second decade and have included more cases in children up to the age of 9, but all agree that most cases are seen before the age of 50. One example recorded by Standish and Shafer was present at birth. Southam found that all but one of the 12 retention cysts in his series were in patients over 50 years. Harrison (1975) analysed 400 mucoceles including 47 of his own cases and the remainder from the literature. He pointed out that extravasation cysts occurred most often in younger patients (84 per cent in first four decades), whereas retention cysts occurred more frequently in older patients (85 per cent older than 40). In my own sample however, 6 of 13 patients with retention cysts were younger than 40.

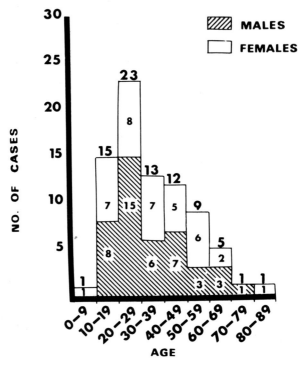

Fig. 98. Age distribution of 80 patients with oral mucoceles.

Sex

In our material, the male : female ratio was 59 : 48 (55 per cent : 45 per cent), which is the same as that reported by Cohen and by Chaudhry et al. In other studies there has been an equal sex incidence.

Race

A substantial majority of our cases occurred in Whites (83 per cent), an observation made also by Standish and Shafer and by Robinson and Hjørting-Hansen.

Site

The great majority of mucoceles are found in the lower lip. In our material, 60 cases (56 per cent) occurred in this site. By comparison, very few occurred in the upper lip (3 per cent). The distribution of the remaining cases is shown in *Table* 8 and is similar to those in other reported series. It may be significant that 6 of the buccal mucosa lesions were retention cysts, representing 37 per cent of the retention cysts. In Harrison's study, 72 per cent of extravasation cysts were found in the lower lip whereas 39 of 40 retention cysts occurred elsewhere in the mouth.

Table 8.
SITE DISTRIBUTION OF 107 MUCOCELES

Site	Number	Percentage
Lower lip	60	56·1
Upper lip	4	3·7
Floor of mouth and ventrum of tongue	15	14·0
Palate	9	8·4
Buccal mucosa	8	7·5
Retromolar	1	0·9
Unspecified	10	9·3
Total	107	99·9

Clinical Presentation
Patients with mucoceles usually complain of a painless swelling which is frequently recurrent. They may have been present for only a few days but some patients tolerate them for months or even years before seeking treatment. The swelling may develop suddenly at mealtimes and many drain spontaneously at intervals. Some 10 per cent of patients are able to relate the development of the cyst to trauma. The mucocele may be only 1–2 mm in diameter but it is usually larger, the majority of them being between 5–10 mm diameter. The ranula is invariably larger than this.

The swellings are round or oval and smooth (*Fig.* 99). The superficial lesions are blue and fluctuant while the deeper lesions are the colour of normal mucosa and are firmer. The superficial cysts give few diagnostic problems but the deeper firmer lesions may be confused with the fibro-epithelial polyp or a small salivary gland tumour. A firm well-demarcated lesion of the upper lip is more likely to be a salivary gland tumour than a mucocele.

Pathogenesis
The pathogenesis of the mucocele has excited a great deal of interest. For many years it was generally believed that obstruction of a salivary duct led to its dilatation proximal to the obstruction, with the formation of an epithelial-lined retention cyst. This concept was questioned by Bhaskar et al. (1956a) who carried out experimental obstruction of the excretory ducts of the submaxillary-sublingual

143

glands in mice over periods ranging from 6 days to 9½ months. They found that mucoceles did not develop although they did find microcyst-like spaces which they believed represented 'tangential cuts through the tortuous dilated ductal elements'. This study was followed by another series of experiments in which the right sub-maxillary excretory ducts of 5 young mice and 6 young rats were exposed and severed. The animals were sacrificed at intervals of from 1 to 9 days postoperatively and the glands were studied grossly

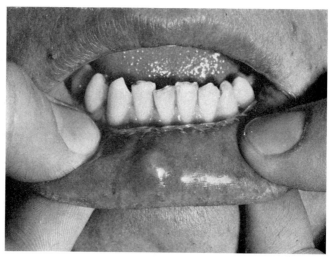

Fig. 99. Mucocele of the lower lip. (*Courtesy of Professor J. J. Pindborg.*)

and microscopically. They found that in 6 of the 9 animals, severing of the duct produced typical mucoceles which were comparable to human lesions. In the early stages there was an accumulation of mucus in the connective tissue and with continuous pooling of saliva a clearly demarcated cavity developed which had no epithelial lining. They concluded that their experiments, when considered with the fact that mucoceles are found most frequently in areas exposed to trauma, such as the lower lip, indicated that a cut or a traumatic defect of a salivary duct was responsible for the production of mucoceles.

The failure to produce mucoceles following acute ligation of the main excretory ducts of the submaxillary and sublingual glands was confirmed experimentally by Standish and Shafer (1957). They did find however that when both the ducts and the arterial blood supply to the glands were ligated, thin-walled dilated ducts of cystic proportions occurred in some 8-, 12- and 16-week animals and

144

appeared to be of submaxillary duct origin. In a later paper Standish and Shafer (1959) reinforced their view that the vast majority of so-called mucous retention cysts represent an extravasation phenomenon in which a ruptured duct allows the ready egress of mucus in the adjacent connective tissue. The smaller number of epithelial-lined mucoceles represent a partial retention phenomenon which is seen as a dilatation of the excretory duct and smaller lobular ducts with concomitant rupture and escape of mucus into the surrounding tissues.

Chaudhry et al. (1960) also concurred with these views but felt that complete severance of the minor salivary glands seemed an impracticable aetiologic factor in the development of human mucoceles and that pinching of the duct seemed to be a more likely explanation for their formation. Their own experimental studies indicated that when the submandibular gland duct of the rat was cut or pinched with a haemostat, mucoceles may be formed by the escape of mucus into the surrounding tissues from the traumatized duct.

Experimental work done on cats (Harrison and Garrett, 1972) has, however, produced results which require that the effects of duct ligation be reappraised. These workers were at pains not to damage the chorda tympani and hence to avoid impairing the para-sympathetic nerve supply to the glands. They therefore investigated the effects of duct ligation of the sublingual salivary gland of the cat. This gland secretes spontaneously, as do the minor salivary glands of man where mucoceles are most frequently found, and has a duct which may readily be tied anterior to the lingual nerve. They found that mucus extravasation occurred in all glands up to 20 days after ligation. Ruptured acini were often observed in the first few days after ligation, but the ducts were not dilated and ductal ruptures were not seen. Ruptured acini were found only very occasionally after 2 days.

The information available at present indicates that most mucoceles in humans probably follow trauma to a duct which is either pinched or severed and this leads to extravasation of mucus. Complete ductal obstruction may lead to the development of a mucous extravasation cyst but this probably occurs less frequently. The rarer mucous retention cyst which is lined by epithelium may possibly, from the very little evidence available, arise in some instances of partial or complete obstruction of the excretory duct by a salivary calculus, by congenital atresia of submandibular duct orifices (Hoggins and Hutton, 1974), or by extraluminal causes. This can lead to dilatation of the duct and also to its rupture.

The presence of eosinophilic oncocyte-like epithelial cells lining some retention cysts of the oral mucosa has led Southam (1974) to postulate that, in the absence of any evidence of duct blockage, these cysts may develop spontaneously in a duct lined by oncocytes. Alternatively, he feels that they may represent a cystic type of papillary cystadenoma.

A third possibility in addition to those of retention and extravasation has been suggested by Praetorius and Hammarström (1974). They believed that those cysts which develop within the gland are caused by trauma to the secretory acinar cells themselves, leading to rupture of these cells and the formation of a mucous pool. They were of the opinion that there need not necessarily be any rupture of the excretory ducts. They call this the 'parenchymatous' type of mucocele.

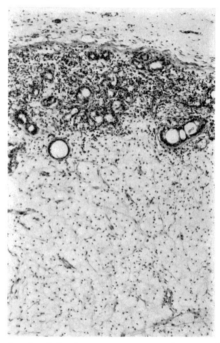

Fig. 100. Poorly defined mucous extravasation cyst filled with muciphages. HE; ×60.

Pathology

Mucoceles are usually received in the laboratory excised with associated salivary gland and frequently a portion of oral mucosa is present on the superficial surface of the lesion. When the specimen is cut the cyst may be discrete, bound by a lining and filled with a gelatinous material. It may also be diffuse and have more liquid mucinous contents.

Histological Features

Microscopically, three distinct morphological patterns have been defined by Robinson and Hjørting-Hansen (1964). Those designated 'poorly-defined cysts' consist of irregularly shaped, poorly-defined pools containing faintly eosinophilic mucinous material and numerous vacuolated macrophages which are sometimes called 'muciphages' (*Fig.* 100). Some of these cysts are small and others extend widely into the connective tissue. There may be communication between the cyst and a duct (*Fig.* 101). Those designated 'well-defined cysts'

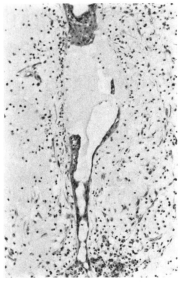

Fig. 101. Ruptured duct with escaping mucus forming an extravasation cyst. HE; ×60.

consist of two groups. Both are sharply circumscribed but they differ in that the periphery of the one consists of granulation tissue or condensed fibrous tissue or both, and is infiltrated by vacuolated macrophages, lymphocytes and polymorphonuclear leucocytes, including eosinophils. One or more dilated ducts may be present and sometimes a breach may be seen in a duct. The second group of well-defined cysts may be partially or completely lined by epithelium. The epithelium varies. It may consist of one or two layers of flattened cells or may be stratified squamous; or the lining may be of one or two layers of cuboidal cells or a thicker pseudostratified columnar epithelium (*Fig.* 102). In their study, Robinson and Hjørting-Hansen were able to demonstrate continuity between

147

a cyst and a duct in 31 of their 150 cases (20 per cent). Granular eosinophilic oncocyte-like cells may be seen in the epithelial linings (Southam, 1974).

Treatment

Mucoceles are best treated by surgical excision including portion of the surrounding tissues. An elliptical incision is made in the mucosa surrounding the cyst which is then dissected with associated mucous glands. The margins of the mucosa are then undermined and sutured in apposition. Attempts to enucleate mucoceles usually fail and recurrences frequently follow.

Small mucoceles may require no surgical treatment provided that the patients find them no hindrance.

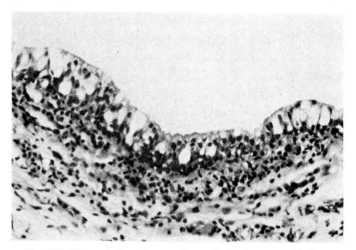

Fig. 102. Mucocele lined by pseudostratified columnar epithelium with goblet cells. HE; ×190.

RANULA

The term 'ranula' is used to describe those mucoceles occurring on the floor of the mouth (*Fig.* 103). They are usually unilateral and because they produce a translucent blue swelling were likened to a frog's belly: from this the term 'ranula' was derived.

Ranulas have been classified as either superficial or plunging. The superficial variety may develop as a retention or extravasation phenomenon associated with trauma to one or more of the numerous excretory ducts of the sublingual salivary gland. Its pathogenesis and pathology are no different from those of the mucoceles elsewhere in the mouth. Significantly, the majority of these ranulas have no epithelial lining.

148

The pathogenesis and treatment of the plunging ranula have been controversial subjects. Roediger and colleagues (1973) have provided evidence to indicate that these ranulas are mucous extravasation cysts of sublingual gland origin which ramify diffusely into the neck.

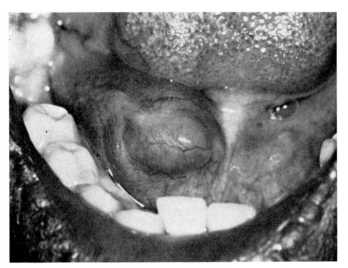

Fig. 103. Ranula.

They recommended surgical removal of the sublingual gland through the mouth without any cervical approach, as the initial form of treatment. They argued that this removes the secreting source, thereby preventing recurrences, and also avoids the problem of a difficult neck dissection.

Congenital sublingual cysts may occur as a result of atresia of the submandibular duct orifices. In the two cases reported by Hoggins and Hutton (1974) it was possible to demonstrate that the cysts were, in fact, dilated submandibular ducts.

149

CHAPTER 17

PARASITIC CYSTS

PARASITIC cysts are rare in the mouth, but hydatid cysts and *Cysticercus cellulosae* are occasionally encountered in the oral tissues.

HYDATID CYST

Hydatid cysts occur in hydatid disease or echinococcosis. There are two species of the genus Echinococcus, *E. granulosus* and *E. multilocularis*. Hydatid disease is caused by the larvae of *E. granulosus*, the dog tapeworm. This tapeworm lives in the intestinal tract of the dog. Its ova are excreted in the faeces of the dog and may be ingested by the intermediate hosts, cattle, sheep and pigs. Man is also a susceptible intermediate host and as dogs are common household pets, may accidentally ingest the ova.

The ingested ova hatch in the upper gastro-intestinal tract from where the small embryos permeate the intestinal mucosa and are dispersed through the blood vessels and lymphatics to all parts of the body. The great majority of cysts are found in the liver, but others are found in the lungs, bones and brain. A few cases have been reported in the tongue. Perl et al. (1972) have described a case in an 18-year-old Black South African woman who complained of a painless swelling on the right side of the tongue which had been present for three months and was increasing in size. An intact unilocular cyst was removed which when cut in half revealed the presence of brood capsules.

The hydatid cysts are initially of microscopic dimensions, but enlarge progressively. The mature cyst consists of three layers, one of host and two of parasitic origin. The host layer consists of fibrous tissue in which there is an infiltrate of chronic inflammatory cells, eosinophils and giant cells. The intermediate layer is white, non-nucleated, and consists of numerous delicate laminations. It usually shrinks away from the outer fibrous layer when the tension within the cyst is relieved. Finally, there is the inner, nucleated germinal layer (*Figs.* 104 and 105). The cyst fluid is relatively clear, albumin-free and contains the so-called 'hydatid sand' consisting of brood capsules and scolices. These brood capsules or daughter cysts develop originally as minute projections of the germinative layer which develop central vesicles and become minute cysts.

Scolices of the head of the worm develop on the inner aspects of the brood capsules. It is when they separate from the germinative layer that they form the 'hydatid sand'.

Hydatid disease is common in sheep-raising countries such as Australia, New Zealand, Argentina and South Africa.

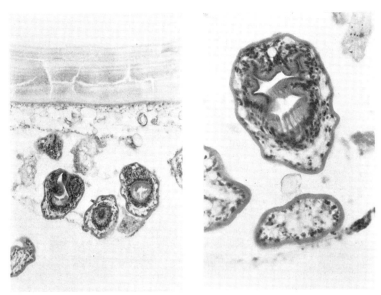

Fig. 104.   Fig. 105.

Fig. 104. Hydatid cyst. Intermediate non-nucleated layer with germinative layer forming brood capsules on its inner aspect. The scolices are formed in these brood capsules. HE; ×125.

Fig. 105. Scolex in the brood capsule of a hydatid cyst. HE; ×325.

CYSTICERCUS CELLULOSAE

Man develops cysticercosis through the larval form, *Cysticercus cellulosae*, of the pork tapeworm *Taenia solium*. He can act as both the intermediate and the definitive host. The adult worm may be ingested in inadequately heated or frozen pork. Alternatively, man may ingest the cysticerci themselves from infested pork and these develop into the adult worm. This lives attached to the wall of the small intestine where, fully grown, it may reach a length of 7 metres. Gravid proglottids or eggs begin to drop off and are passed in the faeces. In this way they may be ingested by man through contaminated food or from their own dirty hands, or they may be regurgitated into the stomach. In the stomach their covering is digested off and the larval forms are hatched. These penetrate the

151

intestinal mucosa and are then distributed through the blood vessels and lymphatics to all parts of the body, where they develop into cysticerci.

There are very few reports of cysticercosis of the oral regions, but Rosencrans and Barak (1969) described a case which involved the lower lip and Timoșca and Gavrili̦ă (1974) have recorded 5 cases in Romanian patients. Two occurred subcutaneously in the neck, two

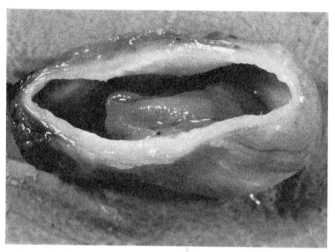

Fig. 106. Gross specimen of *Cysticercus cellulosae* removed from tongue. ×5.

deep to the cheek mucosa and one had multiple lesions involving the lip, cheek and skin. Three examples in the oral tissues have been registered in our files. One occurred as a swelling of the dorsum of the tongue in a 7-year-old child; another in the tongue of a 70-year-old man. The third was a firm mass 10 mm in diameter in the right cheek (Ostrofsky and Baker, 1975). All the specimens were intact cystic masses which, when cut, contained clear watery fluid and a coiled white structure apparently attached to the inner aspect of the cyst (*Fig.* 106).

Histological examination of *Cysticercus cellulosae* shows a dense fibrous outer capsule which is derived from host tissue. This contains a fairly dense inflammatory cell infiltrate consisting predominantly of lymphocytes, plasma cells and histiocytes. On the inner aspect of this fibrous capsule, the nature of the infiltrate is different and consists of a dense aggregation of eosinophil and neutrophil polymorphonuclear leucocytes. A few foci of dystrophic calcification are present in this capsule, and some of these are concentrically laminated. Within the fibrous capsule is a delicate double-layered membrane consisting of an outer acellular hyaline eosinophilic layer and an inner, sparsely cellular layer. This membrane has a loose attachment to the fibrous capsule and is readily

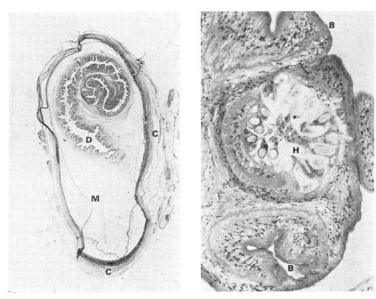

Fig. 107.   Fig. 108.

Fig. 107. *Cysticercus cellulosae* containing the larval form of *Taenia solium*. C, Fibrous outer capsule; M, Double layered membrane; D, Duct-like invagination segment. HE; ×6.

Fig. 108. Scolex of larval form of *Taenia solium*. B, Bothria; H, Hooklets. HE; ×125.

torn away from it. The cyst lies within this membrane and contains the larval form of *T. solium* (*Fig.* 107). At the cephalic extremity of the larva, the scolex with rostellum, bothria (suckers) and hooklets may be identified (*Fig.* 108). Caudal to the scolex is the duct-like invagination segment lined by a homogeneous anhistic membrane.

Although *Cysticercus cellulosae* is harmless in the oral tissues, localization in the brain, heart valves and orbit occurs and produces important functional derangements.

REFERENCES

Abrams A. A. and Howell F. V. (1968) The calcifying odontogenic cyst. *Oral Surg.* **25**, 594–606.

Abrams A. M., Howell F. V. and Bullock W. K. (1963) Nasopalatine cysts. *Oral Surg.* **16**, 306–332.

Ackerman L. V. (1968) *Surgical Pathology*, 4th ed. St. Louis, Mosby, p. 97.

Albers D. D. (1973) Median mandibular cyst partially lined with pseudo-stratified columnar epithelium. *Oral Surg.* **36**, 11–15.

Allison R. T. (1974) Electron microscopic study of 'Rushton' hyaline bodies in cyst linings. *Br. Dent. J.* **137**, 102–104.

Altini M. and Farman A. G. (1975) The calcifying odontogenic cyst. Eight new cases and a review of the literature. *Oral Surg.* **40**, 751–759.

Arey L. B. (1965) *Developmental Anatomy*, 7th ed. Philadelphia and London, Saunders, p. 205.

Arwill T. and Heyden G. (1973) Histochemical studies on cholesterol formation in odontogenic cysts and granulomas. *Scand. J. Dent. Res.* **81**, 406–410.

Bartlett P. F., Radden B. G. and Reade P. C. (1973) The experimental production of odontogenic keratocysts. *J. Oral Pathol.* **2**, 58–67.

Bernier J. L. and Bhaskar S. N. (1958) Aneurysmal bone cysts of the mandible. *Oral Surg.* **11**, 1018–1028.

Bhaskar S. N. (1965) Gingival cysts and the keratinizing ameloblastoma. *Oral Surg.* **19**, 796–807.

Bhaskar S. N. (1966) Lympho-epithelial cysts of the oral cavity. *Oral Surg.* **21**, 120–128.

Bhaskar S. N. (1972) Nonsurgical resolution of radicular cysts. *Oral Surg.* **34**, 458–468.

Bhaskar S. N. and Bernier J. L. (1959) Histogenesis of branchial cysts: a report of 468 cases. *Am. J. Pathol.* **35**, 407–423.

Bhaskar S. N., Bernier J. L. and Godby F. (1959) Aneurysmal bone cyst and other giant cell lesions of the jaws. *J. Oral Surg.* **17**, 30–41.

Bhaskar S. N., Bolden, T. E. and Weinmann J. P. (1956a) Experimental obstructive adenitis in the mouse. *J. Dent. Res.* **35**, 852–862.

Bhaskar S. N., Bolden T. E. and Weinmann J. P. (1956b) Pathogenesis of mucoceles. *J. Dent. Res.* **35**, 863–874.

Binnie W. H. and Rowe A. H. R. (1974) The incidence of epithelial rests, proliferations and apical periodontal cysts following root canal treatment in young dogs. *Br. Dent. J.* **137**, 56–60.

Blair A. E. and Wadsworth W. (1968) Median mandibular developmental cyst. *J. Oral Surg.* **26**, 735–738.

Bouyssou M. and Guilhem A .(1965) Recherches morphologiques et histochimiques sur les corps hyalins intrakystiques de Rushton. *Bull. Group. Int. Rech. Sci. Stomatol.* **8**, 81–104.

Bramley P. A. (1971) Treatment of cysts of the jaws. *Proc. R. Soc. Med.* **64**, 547–550.

REFERENCES

Bramley P. A. (1974) The odontogenic keratocyst—an approach to treatment. *Int. J. Oral Surg.* **3**, 337–341.

Browne R. M. (1969) The pathogenesis of the odontogenic keratocyst. *Fourth Proceedings of the International Academy of Oral Pathology*, p. 28.

Browne R. M. (1970) The odontogenic keratocyst—clinical aspects. *Br. Dent. J.* **128**, 225–231.

Browne R. M. (1971a) The odontogenic keratocyst—histological features and their correlation with clinical behaviour. *Br. Dent. J.* **131**, 249–259.

Browne R. M. (1971b) The origin of cholesterol in odontogenic cysts in man. *Arch. Oral Biol.* **16**, 107–113.

Browne R. M. (1972) Metaplasia and degeneration in odontogenic cysts in man. *J. Oral Pathol.* **1**, 145–158.

Browne R. M. and Gough N. G. (1972) Malignant change in the epithelium lining odontogenic cysts. *Cancer* **29**, 1199–1207.

Buchner A. and Ramon Y. (1974) Median mandibular cyst—A rare lesion of debatable origin. *Oral Surg.* **37**, 431–437.

Burdi A. R. (1968) Distribution of midpalatine cysts—re-evaluation of human palatal closure mechanisms. *J. Oral Surg.* **26**, 41–45.

Burke G. W., Feagans W. M., Elzay R. P. and Schwartz L. D. (1966) Some aspects of the origin and fate of midpalatal cysts in human fetuses. *J. Dent. Res.* **45**, 159–164.

Butz S. (1975) Personal communication.

Byrd D. L., Allen J. W., Kindrick R. D. and De Witt J. D. (1969) Aneurysmal bone cyst of the maxilla. *J. Oral Surg.* **27**, 296–300.

Chaudhry A. P., Reynolds D. H., La Chapelle C. F. and Vickers R. A. (1960) A clinical and experimental study of mucocele (retention cyst). *J. Dent. Res.* **39**, 1253–1262.

Christ T. F. (1970) The globulomaxillary cyst—an embryologic misconception. *Oral Surg.* **30**, 515–526.

Clausen F. P. and Dabelsteen E. (1969) Increase in sensitivity of the rhodamine B method for keratinization by the use of fluorescent light. *Acta Pathol. Microbiol. Scand. (A)* **77**, 169–171.

Clough J. R. and Price C. H. G. (1968) Aneurysmal bone cysts. *J. Bone Joint Surg. (Br.)* **50**, 116–127.

Cohen L. (1965) Mucoceles of the oral cavity. *Oral Surg.* **19**, 365–372.

Courage G. R., North A. F. and Hansen L. S. (1974) Median palatine cysts. Review of the literature and report of a case. *Oral Surg.* **37**, 745–753.

Dabelsteen E. and Fulling H. J. (1971) A preliminary study of blood group substances A and B in oral epithelium exhibiting atypia. *Scand. J. Dent. Res.* **79**, 387–393.

Dascoulis G. (1960) Personal communication.

Daugherty J. W. and Eversole L. R. (1971) Aneurysmal bone cyst of the mandible. Report of a case. *J. Oral Surg.* **29**, 737–741.

Dent R. J. and Wertheimer F. W. (1967) Hyaline bodies in odontogenic cysts—a histochemical study for hemoglobin. *J. Dent. Res.* **46**, 629.

Donoff R. B., Harper E. and Guralnick W. C. (1972) Collagenolytic activity in keratocysts. *J. Oral Surg.* **30**, 879–884.

155

Egyedi P. and Beyazit E. (1973) Marsupialisation of large cysts of the maxilla into the maxillary sinus and/or nose. A follow-up investigation. In: Kay L. W. (ed.) *Oral Surgery IV* (Transactions of the Fourth International Conference on Oral Surgery). Copenhagen, Munksgaard, pp. 81–84.

Emerson T. G., Whitlock R. I. H. and Jones J. H. (1972) Involvement of soft tissue by odontogenic keratocysts (primordial cysts). *Br. J. Oral Surg.* **9**, 181–185.

Ettinger R. L. and Manderson R. D. (1973) Implantation keratinizing epidermoid cysts. *Oral Surg.* **36**, 225–230.

Eversole L. R., Sabes W. R. and Rovin S. (1975) Aggressive growth and neoplastic potential of odontogenic cysts. *Cancer* **35**, 270–282.

Fauchard P. (1746) *The Surgeon Dentist or Treatise on the Teeth* (Tr. Lindsay L. (1946), London, Butterworth, p. 93).

Fejerskov O. and Krogh J. (1972) The calcifying ghost cell odontogenic tumor—or the calcifying odontogenic cyst. *J. Oral Pathol.* **1**, 273–287.

Fell H. (1957) The effect of excess vitamin A on cultures of embryonic chicken skin explanted at different stages of differentiation. *Proc. R. Soc. Lond. (Biol.)* **146**, 242–256.

Ferenczy K. (1958) The relationship of globulomaxillary cysts to the fusion of embryonal processes and to cleft palates. *Oral Surg.* **11**, 1388–1393.

Fickling B. W. (1965) Cysts of the jaw—a long term survey of types and treatment. *Proc. R. Soc. Med.* **58**, 847–854.

Fink H. A. (1963) Retention cyst of the tongue. *Oral Surg.* **16**, 1290–1293.

Fløe Møller J. and Philipsen H. P. (1958) Et tilfaelde af nasoalveolaer cyste (Klestadt's cyste). A case of nasoalveolar cyst (Klestadt's cyst). *Tandlaegebladet* **62**, 659–668.

Fordyce G. L. (1956) The probable nature of so-called latent haemorrhagic cysts of the mandible. *Br. Dent. J.* **101**, 40–42.

Frithiof L. and Hägglund G. (1966) Ultrastructure of the capsular epithelium of radicular cysts. *Acta Odontol. Scand.* **24**, 23–34.

Fromm A. (1967) Epstein's pearls, Bohn's nodules and inclusion cysts of the oral cavity. *J. Dent. Child.* **34**, 275.

Gardner A. F., Gallagher C. A. and Glaser R. I. (1963) The life history of the oral mucocele. *Northwest Dent.* **42**, 103–107.

Gillette R. and Weinmann J. P. (1958) Extrafollicular stages in dentigerous cyst development. *Oral Surg.* **11**, 638–645.

Giunta J. and Cataldo E. (1973) Lympho-epithelial cysts of the oral mucosa. *Oral Surg.* **35**, 77–84.

Gold L. and Sliwkowski A. S. (1973) Lateral periodontal cyst—a clinical and histological study. In: Kay L. W. (ed.) *Oral Surgery IV* (Transactions of the Fourth International Conference on Oral Surgery). Copenhagen, Munksgaard, pp. 85–89.

Gorlin R. J. (1957) Potentialities of oral epithelium manifest by mandibular dentigerous cysts. *Oral Surg.* **10**, 271–284.

Gorlin R. J. and Goltz R. W. (1960) Multiple nevoid basal cell epithelioma, jaw cysts and bifid rib: a syndrome. *N. Engl. J. Med.* **262**, 908–912.

Gorlin R. J. and Jirasek J. E. (1970) Oral cysts containing gastric or intestinal mucosa—unusual embryologic accident or heterotopia. *J. Oral Surg.* **28**, 9–11.

Gorlin R. J., Pindborg J. J., Clausen F. P. and Vickers R. A. (1962) The calcifying odontogenic cyst—a possible analogue of the cutaneous calcifying epithelioma of Malherbe. *Oral Surg.* **15**, 1235–1243.

Gorlin R. J., Pindborg J. J., Redman R. S., Williamson J. J. and Hansen L. S. (1964) The calcifying odontogenic cyst. A new entity and possible analogue of the cutaneous calcifying epithelioma of Malherbe. *Cancer* **17**, 723–729.

Grand N. G. and Marwah A. S. (1964) Pigmented gingival cyst. *Oral Surg.* **17**, 635–639.

Gregory G. T. and Shafer W. G. (1958) Surgical ciliated cysts of the maxilla. *J. Oral Surg.* **16**, 251–253.

Grupe H. E., jun., Ten Cate A. R. and Zander H. A. (1967) A histochemical and radiobiological study of in vitro and in vivo human epithelial cell rest proliferation. *Arch. Oral Biol.* **12**, 1321–1329.

Gruskin S. E. and Dahlin D. C. (1968) Aneurysmal bone cysts of the jaws. *J. Oral Surg.* **26**, 523–528.

Hamilton W. J. and Mossman H. W. (1972) *Human Embryology*, 4th ed. Cambridge, Heffer, p. 302.

Hansen J. (1967) Keratocysts in the jaws. In: Husted E. and Hjørting-Hansen E. (ed.) *Oral Surgery II* (Transactions of the Second International Conference on Oral Surgery). Copenhagen, Munksgaard, pp. 128–134.

Hansen J. and Kobayasi T. (1970a) Ultrastructural studies of odontogenic cysts—I. Non-keratinizing cysts. *Acta Morphol. Neerl. Scand.* **8**, 29–42.

Hansen J. and Kobayasi T. (1970b) Ultrastructural studies of odontogenic cysts—II. Keratinizing cysts. *Acta Morphol. Neerl. Scand.* **8**, 43–62.

Hansen L. S., Sapone J. and Sproat R. C. (1974) Traumatic bone cysts of jaws. *Oral Surg.* **37**, 899–910.

Harris M. and Goldhaber P. (1973) The production of a bone resorbing factor by dental cysts in vitro. *Br. J. Oral Surg.* **10**, 334–338.

Harris M., Jenkins M. V., Bennett A. and Wills M. R. (1973) Prostaglandin production and bone resorption by dental cysts. *Nature* **245**, 213–215.

Harrison J. D. (1975) Salivary mucoceles. *Oral Surg.* **39**, 268–278.

Harrison J. D. and Garrett J. R. (1972) Mucocele formation in cats by glandular duct ligation. *Arch. Oral Biol.* **17**, 1403–1414.

Harvey S. H. (1855) Tumours caused by carious tooth. *Am. J. Dent. Surg.* **2**, 589–590.

Heath C. (1880) Thirty-five-years history of a maxillary tumour. *Br. J. Dent. Sci.* **23**, 502–505.

Heath C. (1887) Cystic diseases of the jaws. *Br. J. Dent.* **8**, 615–626, 422–434.

Hjørting-Hansen E. (1970) *Studies on Implantation of an Organic Bone in Cystic Jaw Lesions.* Copenhagen, Munksgaard.

Hjørting-Hansen E., Andreasen J. O. and Robinson L. H. (1969) A study of odontogenic cysts with special reference to location of keratocysts. *Br. J. Oral Surg.* **7**, 15–23.

Hodson J. J. (1962) Epithelial residues of the jaw with special reference to the edentulous jaw. *J. Anat.* **96**, 16–24.

Hoggins G. S. and Hutton J. B. (1974) Congenital sublingual cystic swellings due to imperforate salivary ducts. *Oral Surg.* **37**, 370–373.

Howe G. L. (1965) 'Haemorrhagic cysts' of the mandible. *Br. J. Oral Surg.* **3**, 55–75, 77–91.

Huebner G. R. and Turlington E. G. (1971) So-called traumatic (haemorrhagic) bone cysts of the jaws. *Oral Surg.* **31**, 354–365.

Hunter J. (1780) Quoted from Palmer J. F. (ed.) (1835) *The Works of John Hunter F.R.S. with Notes.* London, Longman, vol. 1, p. 70.

Issa M. A. and Davies J. D. (1971) Dermoid cyst of the jaw. *Br. Dent. J.* **131**, 543–546.

Jacobson A. (1967) The Bantu Dentition. Ph.D. thesis, University of the Witwatersrand, Johannesburg, p. 26.

Jaffe H. L. and Lichtenstein L. (1942) Solitary unicameral bone cyst with emphasis on the roentgen picture, the pathologic appearance, and the pathogenesis. *Arch. Surg.* **44**, 1004.

Jensen J. L. and Erickson J. O. (1974) Hyaline bodies in odontogenic cysts: Electron microscopic observations. *J. Oral Pathol.* **3**, 1–6.

Kay L. W. and Kramer I. R. H. (1962) Squamous cell carcinoma arising in a dental cyst. *Oral Surg.* **15**, 970–979.

Killey H. C. and Kay L. W. (1972) *Benign Cystic Lesions of the Jaws, their Diagnosis and Treatment*, 2nd ed. Edinburgh and London, Churchill Livingstone.

Killey H. C. and Kay L. W. (1973) Benign mucosal cysts. In: Kay L. W. (ed.) *Oral Surgery IV* (Transactions of the Fourth International Conference on Oral Surgery). Copenhagen, Munksgaard, pp. 169–174.

Kramer I. R. H. (1963) Ameloblastoma: A clinicopathological appraisal. *Br. J. Oral Surg.* **1**, 13–28.

Kramer I. R. H. (1970) Letter to the editor on 'the odontogenic keratocyst'. *Br. Dent. J.* **128**, 370.

Kramer I. R. H. (1974) Changing views on oral disease. *Proc. R. Soc. Med.* **67**, 271–276.

Kramer I. R. H. and Toller P. A. (1973) The use of exfoliative cytology and protein estimations in preoperative diagnosis of odontogenic keratocysts. *Int. J. Oral Surg.* **2**, 143–151.

Kwapis B. W. and Whitten J. B. (1971) Mucosal cysts of the maxillary sinus. *J. Oral Surg.* **29**, 561–566.

Little J. W. and Jakobsen J. (1973) Origin of the globulomaxillary cyst. *J. Oral Surg.* **31**, 188–195.

Livingston A. (1927) Observations on the development of the dental cyst. *Dent. Record* **47**, 531–538.

Lucas R. B. (1954) Neoplasia in odontogenic cysts. *Oral Surg.* **7**, 1227–1235.

Lucas R. B. (1972) *Pathology of Tumours of the Oral Tissues*, 2nd ed. Edinburgh and London, Churchill Livingstone.

Lucchesi F. J. and Topazian D. S. (1961) Multilocular median developmental cysts of the mandible. *J. Oral Surg.* **19**, 336–338.

Lufkin A. W. (1938) *History of Dentistry*. London, Kimpton, p. 60.

REFERENCES

Lundström A. (1960) *Introduction to Orthodontics.* New York, Toronto and London, McGraw-Hill, Ch. 8, pp. 150–151.

Lutz J., Cimasoni G. and Held A. J. (1965) Histochemical observations on the epithelial lining of radicular cysts. *Acta Odontol. Scand.* **9**, 90–95.

Main D. M. G. (1970a) Epithelial jaw cysts: a clinicopathological reappraisal. *Br. J. Oral Surg.* **8**, 114–125.

Main D. M. G. (1970b) The enlargement of epithelial jaw cysts. *Odontol. Revy* **21**, 29–49.

Mayer R., Libotte M. and Ruppol P. (1967) La lacune essentielle de la mandibule. *Acta Stomatol. Belg.* **64**, 33–52.

Meerkotter V. (1969) The ameloblastoma in the Witwatersrand area. *Fourth Proceedings of the International Academy of Oral Pathology,* p. 144.

Meyer I. (1955) Dermoid cysts (dermoids) of the floor of the mouth. *Oral Surg,* **8**, 1149–1164.

Meyer I. (1957) Developmental median cyst of the mandible. *Oral Surg.* **10**, 75–80.

Monteleone L. and McLellan M. S. (1964) Epstein's pearls (Bohn's nodules) of the palate. *J. Oral Surg.* **22**, 301–304.

Moon (1877–1878) Radicular odontome. *Odontol. Soc. Trans.* 2nd series, **10**, 30–31.

Morgan P. R. and Heyden G. (1975) Enzyme histochemical studies on the formation of hyalin bodies in the epithelium of odontogenic cysts. *J. Oral Pathol.* **4**, 120–127.

Morgan P. R. and Johnson N. W. (1974) Histological, histochemical and ultrastructural studies on the nature of hyalin bodies in odontogenic cysts. *J. Oral Pathol.* **3**, 127–147.

Mortensen H., Winther J. E. and Birn H. (1970) Periapical granulomas and cysts. An investigation of 1600 cases. *Scand. J. Dent. Res.* **78**, 241–250.

Moskow B. S. (1966) The pathogenesis of the gingival cyst. *Periodontics* **4**, 23–28.

Moskow B. S., Siegel K., Zegarelli E. V., Kutscher A. H. and Rothenberg F. (1970) Gingival and lateral periodontal cysts. *J. Periodontol.* **41**, 249–260.

Mourshed F. (1964a) A roentgenographic study of dentigerous cysts. I.—Incidence in a population sample. *Oral Surg.* **18**, 47–53.

Mourshed F. (1964b) A roentgenographic study of dentigerous cysts. II.—Role of roentgenograms in detecting dentigerous cyst in the early stages. *Oral Surg.* **18**, 54–61.

Mourshed F. (1964c) A roentgenographic study of dentigerous cysts. III.—Analysis of 180 cases. *Oral Surg.* **18**, 466–473.

Myall R. W. T., Eastep P. B. and Silver J. G. (1974) Mucous retention cysts of the maxillary antrum. *J. Am. Dent. Assoc.* **89**, 1338–1342.

Oehlers F. A. C. (1970) Periapical lesions and residual dental cysts. *Br. J. Oral Surg.* **8**, 103–113.

Olech E. (1957) Median mandibular cysts. *Oral Surg.* **10**, 69–74.

Olech E., Sicher H. and Weinmann J. P. (1951) Traumatic mandibular bone cysts. *Oral Surg.* **4**, 1160–1172.

159

Oliver L. P. (1973) Aneurysmal bone cyst—Report of a case. *Oral Surg.* 35, 67–76.

Ostrofsky M. K. and Baker M. A. A. (1975) Oral cysticercosis. *J. Dent. Assoc. S. Afr.* 30, 535–537.

Panders A. K. and Hadders H. N. (1969) Solitary keratocysts of the jaws. *J. Oral Surg.* 26, 931–938.

Patten B. M. (1961) The Normal Development of the Facial Region. In: Prizansky S. (ed.) *Congenital Anomalies of the Face and Associated Structures.* Springfield, Thomas, pp. 11–45. (Quoted by Little and Jakobsen, 1973.)

Payne T. F. (1972) An analysis of the clinical and histopathologic parameters of the odontogenic keratocyst. *Oral Surg.* 33, 538–546.

Pedley N. (1886) Cyst of the upper jaw. *Br. Dent. Ass. J.* 7, 289.

Perl P., Perl T. and Goldberg B. (1972) Hydatid cyst in the tongue. *Oral Surg.* 33, 579–581.

Philipsen H. P. (1956) Om keratocyster (kolesteatom) i kaeberne. *Tandlaegebladet* 60, 963–981.

Pindborg J. J. and Hansen J. (1963) Studies on odontogenic cyst epithelium. 2. Clinical and roentgenologic aspects of odontogenic keratocysts. *Acta Pathol. Microbiol. Scand. (A)* 58, 283–294.

Pindborg J. J. and Hjørting-Hansen E. (1974) *Atlas of Diseases of the Jaws,* 1st ed. Copenhagen, Munksgaard.

Pindborg J. J. and Kramer I. R. H. (1971) *Histological Typing of Odontogenic Tumours, Jaw Cysts, and Allied Lesions.* Geneva, World Health Organization.

Pindborg J. J., Philipsen H. P. and Henriksen J. (1962) Studies on odontogenic cyst epithelium—keratinization in odontogenic cysts. In: *Fundamentals of Keratinization.* Washington D.C., American Association for the Advancement of Science, p. 151.

Poyton H. G. and Morgan G. A. (1965) The simple bone cyst. *Oral Surg.* 20, 188–197.

Praetorius F. (1975) Calcifying odontogenic cyst: range, variations and neoplastic potential. Paper delivered at a Symposium on Maxillo-facial Bone Pathology, Brussels, 30–31 March, 1974, organized by Committee on Maxillo-facial Bone Pathology. *Int. J. Oral Surg.* 4, 89 (Abstr.).

Praetorius F. and Hammarström L. (1974) A new concept of the pathogenesis of oral mucous cysts based upon a study of 200 cysts. Personal communication.

Quinn J. H. (1960) Congenital epidermoid cyst of anterior half of tongue. *Oral Surg.* 13, 1283–1287.

Radden B. G. and Reade P. C. (1973) Odontogenic cysts. A review and clinicopathological study of 368 odontogenic cysts. *Aust. Dent. J.* 18, 218–225.

Rickles N. H. and Little J. W. (1967) The histogenesis of the branchial cyst. *Am. J. Pathol.* 40, 533–547.

Ritchey B. and Orban B. (1953) Cysts of the gingivae. *Oral Surg.* 6, 765–771.

Riviere G. R. and Sabet T. Y. (1973) Experimental follicular cysts in mice—A histologic study. *Oral Surg.* 36, 205–213.

Robinson L. and Hjørting-Hansen E. (1964) Pathologic changes associated with mucous retention cysts of minor salivary glands. *Oral Surg.* **18**, 191–205.

Roediger W. E. W., Lloyd P. and Lawson H. H. (1973) Mucous extravasation theory as a cause of plunging ranulas. *Br. J. Surg.* **60**, 720–722.

Roed-Petersen B. (1969) Nasolabial cysts. *Br. J. Oral Surg.* **7**, 84–95.

Roper-Hall H. T. (1938) Cysts of developmental origin in the premaxillary region, with special reference to their diagnosis. *Br. Dent. J.* **65**, 405–436.

Rosencrans M. and Barak J. (1969) Parasitic infection of the mouth—A case report of cysticercus cellulosae. *N. Y. State Dent. J.* **35**, 271–273.

Rud J. and Pindborg J. J. (1969) Odontogenic keratocysts: a follow-up study of 21 cases. *J. Oral Surg.* **27**, 323–330.

Ruffer M. A. (1921) *Studies in the Palaeopathology of Egypt.* (Ed. Moodie R. L.) Chicago, University of Chicago Press.

Rushton M. A. (1955) Hyaline bodies in the epithelium of dental cysts. *Proc. R. Soc. Med.* **48**, 407–409.

Salama N. and Hilmy A. (1951) Ancient Egyptian skull and a mandible showing cysts. *Br. Dent. J.* **90**, 17–18.

Saunders I. D. F. (1972) Bohn's nodules—a case report. *Br. Dent. J.* **132**, 457–458.

Schiødt M. and Friis-Hasché E. (1972) Fire tilfaede af oral lymfo-epiteliale cyster. *Tandlaegebladet* **76**, 1075–1081.

Sedano H. O. and Gorlin R. J. (1968) Hyaline bodies of Rushton; some histochemical considerations concerning their etiology. *Oral Surg.* **26**, 198–201.

Seward G. R. (1962) Naso-labial cysts and their radiology. *Dent. Pract.* **12**, 154–161.

Seward G. R. (1964) *Radiology in General Dental Practice.* London, British Dental Association.

Seward G. R. (1965) Dermoid cysts of the floor of the mouth. *Br. J. Oral Surg.* **3**, 36–47.

Seward M. H. (1973) Eruption cyst: an analysis of its clinical features. *J. Oral Surg.* **31**, 31–35.

Sewerin I. and Praetorius F. (1974) Keratin-filled pseudocysts of ducts of sebaceous glands of the vermilion border of the lip. *J. Oral Pathol.* **3**, 279–283.

Shafer W. G., Hine M. K. and Levy B. M. (1974) *A Textbook of Oral Pathology*, 3rd ed. Philadelphia and London, Saunders.

Shear M. (1960a) Primordial cysts. *J. Dent. Assoc. S. Afr.* **15**, 211–217.

Shear M. (1960b) Secretory epithelium in the lining of dental cysts. *J. Dent. Assoc. S. Afr.* **15**, 117–122.

Shear M. (1961a) Clinical statistics of dental cysts. *J. Dent. Assoc. S. Afr.* **16**, 360–364.

Shear M. (1961b) The hyaline and granular bodies in dental cysts. *Br. Dent. J.* **110**, 301–307.

Shear M. (1963a) The histogenesis of the dental cyst. *Dent. Pract.* **13**, 238–243.

Shear M. (1963b) Cholesterol in dental cysts. *Oral Surg.* **16**, 1465–1473.

Shear M. (1963c) The microscopic features of the fibrous walls of dental cysts. *Diastema* **1**, 9–13.

Shear M. (1964) Inflammation in dental cysts. *Oral Surg.* **17**, 756–767.

Shear M. and Pindborg J. J. (1975) Microscopic features of the lateral periodontal cyst. *Scand. J. Dent. Res.* **83**, 103–110.

Sicher H. (1962) Anatomy and oral pathology. *Oral Surg.* **15**, 1264–1269.

Skaug N. (1973) Proteins in fluid from non-keratinizing jaw cysts. *J. Oral Pathol.* **2**, 280–291.

Skaug N. (1974) Proteins in fluid from non-keratinizing jaw cysts. 4. Concentrations of immunoglobulins (IgG, IgA and IgM) and some non-immunoglobulin proteins—Relevance to concepts of cyst wall permeability and clearance of cystic proteins. *J. Oral Pathol.* **3**, 47–61.

Soskolne W. A. and Shear M. (1967) Observations on the pathogenesis of primordial cysts. *Br. Dent. J.* **123**, 321–326.

Southam J. C. (1974) Retention mucoceles of the oral mucosa. *J. Oral Pathol.* **3**, 197–202.

Spence C. B. (1853–4) Diseases of the surrounding tissues originating in carious teeth. *Am. J. Dent. Surg.* 2nd series, 278–282.

Spouge J. D. (1966) Sebaceous metaplasia in the oral cavity occurring in association with dentigerous cyst epithelium. *Oral Surg.* **21**, 492–498.

Stafne E. C. (1942) Bone cavities situated near the angle of the mandible. *J. Am. Dent. Assoc.* **29**, 1969–1972.

Stafne E. C. (1969) *Oral Roentgenographic Diagnosis*, 3rd ed. Philadelphia and London, Saunders, p. 159.

Standish S. M. and Shafer W. G. (1957) Serial histologic effects of rat submaxillary and sublingual gland duct and blood vessel ligation. *J. Dent. Res.* **36**, 866–879.

Standish S. M. and Shafer W. G. (1958) The lateral periodontal cyst. *J. Periodontol.* **29**, 27–33.

Standish S. M. and Shafer W. G. (1959) The mucous retention phenomenon. *J. Oral Surg.* **17**, 15–22.

Stanley H. R., Krogh H. and Pannuk E. (1965) Age changes in the epithelial components of follicles (dental sacs) associated with impacted third molars. *Oral Surg.* **19**, 128–139.

Stoelinga P. J. W. (1971) Over kaak-kysten. M.D. thesis, University of Nijmegen. Nijmegen, Centrale Drukkerij N.V.

Stoelinga P. J. W. (1973) Recurrences and multiplicity of cysts. In: Kay L. W. (ed.) *Oral Surgery IV* (Transactions of the Fourth International Conference on Oral Surgery). Copenhagen, Munksgaard, pp. 77–80.

Stoelinga P. J. W. and Peters J. H. (1973) A note on the origin of keratocysts of the jaws. *Int. J. Oral Surg.* **2**, 37–44.

Stout F. W., Lunin M. and Calonius P. E. B. (1968) A study of epithelial remnants in the maxilla. *Abstracts of the 46th General Meeting of the International Association for Dental Research.* Abstracts 419, 420, 421, pp. 142–143.

Struthers P. and Shear M. (1976) Root resorption produced by the enlargement of ameloblastomas and cysts of the jaws. *Int. J. Oral Surg.* **5**, in the press.

REFERENCES

Summers L. (1972) Cavitation of apical cysts. *J. Dent. Res.* **51**, 1247.
Summers L. (1974) The incidence of epithelium in periapical granulomas and the mechanism of cavitation in apical dental cysts in man. *Arch. Oral Biol.* **19**, 1177–1180.
Ten Cate A. R. (1972) The epithelial cell rests of Malassez and the genesis of the dental cyst. *Oral Surg.* **34**, 956–964.
Thoma K. (1937) Facial cleft or fissural cyst. *Int. J. Orthod.* **23**, 83–89.
Timoşca G. and Gavriliţă L. (1974) Cysticercosis of the maxillofacial region. *Oral Surg.* **37**, 390–400.
Toller P. A. (1948) Experimental investigations into factors concerning the growth of cysts of the jaws. *Proc. R. Soc. Med.* **41**, 681–688.
Toller P. A. (1964) Radioactive isotope and other investigations in a case of haemorrhagic cyst of the mandible. *Br. J. Oral Surg.* **2**, 86–93.
Toller P. A. (1966a) Epithelial discontinuities in cysts of the jaws. *Br. Dent. J.* **120**, 74–78.
Toller P. A. (1966b) Permeability of cyst walls in vivo: investigations with radioactive tracers. *Proc. R. Soc. Med.* **59**, 724–729.
Toller P. A. (1967) Origin and growth of cysts of the jaws. *Ann. R. Coll. Surg. Engl.* **40**, 306–336.
Toller P. A. (1970a) Protein substances in odontogenic cyst fluids. *Br. Dent. J.* **128**, 317–322.
Toller P. A. (1970b) The osmolality of fluids from cysts of the jaws. *Br. Dent. J.* **129**, 275–278.
Toller P. A. (1971) Autoradiography of explants from odontogenic cysts. *Br. Dent. J.* **131**, 57–61.
Toller P. A. (1972) Newer concepts of odontogenic cysts. *Int. J. Oral Surg.* **1**, 3–16.
Toller P. A. and Holborow E. J. (1969) Immunoglobulins and immunoglobulin-containing cells in cysts of the jaws. *Lancet* **2**, 178.
Tolman D. E. and Stafne E. C. (1967) Developmental bone defects of the mandible. *Oral Surg.* **24**, 488–490.
Traeger K. A. (1961) Cyst of the gingiva (mucocele): report of a case. *Oral Surg.* **14**, 243–245.
Trott J. R., Chebib F. and Galindo Y. (1973) Factors related to cholesterol formation in cysts and granulomas. *J. Can. Dent. Assoc.* **39**, 550–555.
Trott J. R. and Esty C. (1972) An analysis of 105 dental cysts. *J. Can. Dent. Assoc.* **38**, 75–78.
Ulmansky M., Azaz B. and Sela J. (1969) Calcifying odontogenic cyst. *J. Oral Surg.* **27**, 415–419.
Valderhaug J. (1974) A histologic study of experimentally induced periapical inflammation in primary teeth in monkeys. *Int. J. Oral Surg.* **3**, 111–113.
Van Doorn M. E. (1972) Enucleation and primary closure of jaw cysts. *Int. J. Oral Surg.* **1**, 17–25.
Vedtofte P. and Dabelsteen E. (1975) Blood group antigens A and B in ameloblastomas, odontogenic keratocysts and nonkeratinizing cysts. *Scand. J. Dent. Res.* **83**, 96–102.

Vickers R. A. and von der Muhll O. H. (1966) An investigation concerning inducibility of lymphoepithelial cysts in hamsters by autogenous epithelial transplantation. *J. Dent. Res.* **45**, 1029–1032.

Waldron C. A. (1969) Some observations on the jaw cysts in the basal cell nevoid carcinoma syndrome. *Fourth Proceedings of the International Academy of Oral Pathology*, p. 220.

Ward T. G. and Cohen B. (1963) Squamous carcinoma in a mandibular cyst. *Br. J. Oral Surg.* **1**, 8–12.

Warwick R. and Williams P. L. (ed.) (1973) *Gray's Anatomy*, 35th ed. London, Longman, p. 116.

Weathers D. R. and Waldron C. A. (1973) Unusual multilocular cysts of the jaws (botryoid odontogenic cysts). *Oral Surg.* **36**, 235–241.

Wertheimer F. W., Fullmer H. M. and Hansen L. S. (1962) A histochemical study of hyaline bodies in odontogenic cysts and a comparison to the human secondary dental cuticle. *Oral Surg.* **15**, 1466.

Zegarelli D. J. and Zegarelli E. V. (1973) Radiolucent lesions in the globulomaxillary region. *J. Oral Surg.* **31**, 767–771.

INDEX

Kafedžiūke violetą

... M ujoj neme svoje blepo sloze ...